IMMUNOPATHOGENESIS AND IMMUNE-BASED THERAPY FOR SELECTED AUTOIMMUNE DISORDERS

Edited by **Mourad Aribi**

Immunopathogenesis and Immune-based Therapy for Selected Autoimmune Disorders
http://dx.doi.org/10.5772/63032
Edited by Mourad Aribi

Contributors

Kouichi Hirayama, Miho Nagai, Eleonora Kurtenbach, Camila Guerra Martinez, Kokil Tandon, Denise Faustman, Miriam Davis, Willem M. Kuhtreiber, Mark Russell, Nidhi Sofat, Anna Pituch-Noworolska, Monika Mach-Tomalska, Jianxun Song, Mohammad Haque, Praneet Sandhu, Swetha Ravi, Sravya Kurapati, Mourad Aribi

Published by InTech
Janeza Trdine 9, 51000 Rijeka, Croatia

Publishing Process Manager Martina Usljebrka
Technical Editor SPi Global
Cover InTech Design team

First published March, 2017
Printed in Croatia
Legal deposit, Croatia: National and University Library in Zagreb

Additional hard copies can be obtained from orders@intechopen.com

Immunopathogenesis and Immune-based Therapy for Selected Autoimmune Disorders, Edited by Mourad Aribi
p. cm.
Print ISBN 978-953-51-3021-5
Online ISBN 978-953-51-3022-2

For EU product safety concerns:
IN TECH d.o.o., Prolaz Marije Krucifikse Kozulić 3, 51000 Rijeka, Croatia,
info@intechopen.com or visit our website at intechopen.com.

Meet the editor

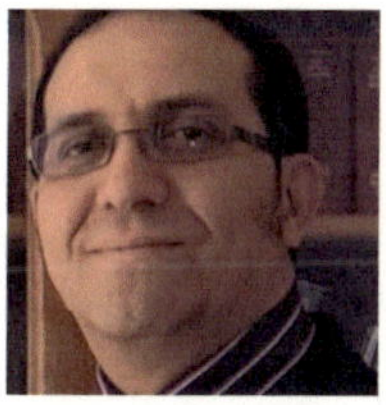

Dr. Mourad Aribi, PhD, Dr. Hab., is a professor of Immunology at the University of Tlemcen (Algeria). He is also the founder and director of the Laboratory of Applied Molecular Biology and Immunology. His current research focuses on the modulation of cell-mediated and inflammatory immune responses in autoimmune diseases, cancer diseases, and infectious diseases. Thanks to his interdisciplinary skills, he was able to develop numerous high-level collaboration projects, notably with CNRS and INSERM partners (CNRS UPR 1142, University of Montpellier; INSERM U1090, Luminy, Aix-Marseille University; and INSERM U866, Burgundy, France). He is a reviewer in several international journals and is also a member of the Editorial Board of *Frontiers in Immunology* (the official journal of the International Union of Immunological Societies, IUIS).

Contents

Preface

This book is a synthesis work that discusses two main aspects of autoimmunity: immunopathogenesis and therapeutic approaches essentially based on the immunotherapies.

It consists of eight chapters, beginning with an Introductory Chapter dedicated to give a global view on the immune system and autoimmune diseases, deliberately in a succinct way.

Chapter 2 discusses how antigen-specific regulatory T cells (Tregs) can be generated from pluripotent stem cells and their ability to reduce blood glucose level in a mouse model of type 1 diabetes.

Chapter 3 focuses more specifically on the analysis of the differences between early- and late-onset type 1 diabetes by concentrating upon three key points: C-peptide detection and levels, persistence of autoreactive T cells, and differences in metabolites.

The main purpose of Chapter 4 is to show the roles of both cytokines interferon-gamma (IFN-γ) and interleukin-17 (IL-17) that seem to have opposing effects in autoimmune cardiomyopathy.

Chapter 5 aims to review mechanisms of autoimmunity and immunotherapy of gastrointestinal tract.

The purpose of Chapter 6 is to suggest systemic sclerosis as an example of how research into pathogenic processes can be translated into novel therapeutic targets for autoimmune conditions.

Chapter 7 discusses both the clinical and immunological aspects of myasthenia gravis and its subgroups based on its characterization of the antigenic targets.

Chapter 8 reviews autoimmune anomalies associated with the increased expression of B cell–activating factor of the tumour necrosis factor family (BAFF), also known as B lymphocyte stimulator (BLyS), and anti-BAFF therapy in autoimmune diseases.

As you will see, the goal of most of these chapters is not to give details on the entire architecture of autoimmune diseases but rather to tackle specific questions on the immunopathogenic mechanisms and/or immunotherapeutic approaches of a number of autoimmune disorders, including type 1 diabetes, autoimmune cardiomyopathy, autoimmunity of gastrointestinal tract, systemic sclerosis, and myasthenia gravis.

I really hope that these chapters will be useful and informative for clinicians, biologists, researchers, teachers, and students who are interested in immunology and immunopathology.

I would like to thank all the collaborators who had accepted to participate in making this book which would not see the light also without devoted work of Martina Usljebrka, Publishing Process Manager. I would like to thank her and thank all the team of InTech Publishing House, for their trust, their patience, and their help in making this book.

Prof. Mourad Aribi
Laboratory of Applied Molecular Biology and Immunology
University of Tlemcen, Algeria

Chapter 1

Introductory Chapter: Immune System Dysfunction and Autoimmune Diseases

Mourad Aribi

Additional information is available at the end of the chapter

http://dx.doi.org/10.5772/67671

1. Introduction

Currently, a major health concern is focused on many diseases caused by heterogeneous aberrations of the immune system, including autoimmune diseases, which account for one of the top leading causes of death worldwide. The molecular approach has provided an answer to several fundamental questions about the etiopathogenetic mechanisms of such diseases and has thus considerably provided the opportunity for researchers and clinicians to compare their own experiences and to bring their hypotheses closer together. It therefore appears appropriate to propose this collective work, which contains various and often specific subjects on autoimmune disorders.

2. Immune system: self- and non–self-discrimination

The essential functions of the immune system is to maintain the coherence of the cells and tissues and to ensure their integrity by rejecting foreign aggressive substances or infectious agents, that is, the "nonself," and the immunogenic altered self, referred to as "modified self," while respecting the normal components of the host, that is, the "unmodified self-antigens" [1, 2] (**Figure 1**).

Two strategies are adopted to preserve immune system integrity and coherence [3]: the first strategy corresponds to the innate immunity, also known as nonadaptive immunity, which is triggered immediately after infiltration of microorganisms or upon danger signal integration; the second one involves adaptive immunity, which the activation takes place after pretreatment of the antigen by innate immune cells. Adaptive immunity develops more slowly than innate immunity. It is characterized by immunological memory, allowing it to generate faster and more intense responses in subsequent exposures to the same antigen, which has previously induced a primary immune response.

Cells of innate immunity can recognize, through membrane or intracellular genetically encoded receptors (pattern recognition receptors, PRRs), invariant motifs (pathogen-associated molecular patterns, PAMPs) that are displayed on a large number of pathogens, but absent in host cells. These receptors are preformed or very rapidly inducible in humans. They

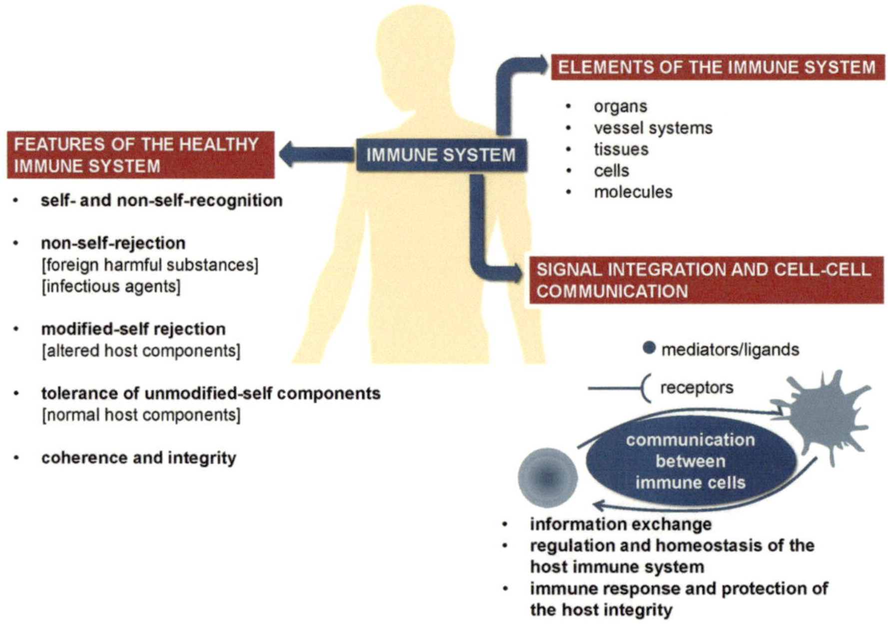

Figure 1. Overview of the immune system. The immune system contains a complex collection of organs, tissues and vessel systems between which circulate constantly immunocompetent cells of innate and adaptive immunity. These cells communicate with each other via receptors that integrate external signals in the form of soluble mediators or insoluble extracellular ligands or counterreceptors. The binding of a signal induces a transformation of the external information into internal information, a process referred to as a signal transduction inside the cell, and a modification of the properties of the molecular targets involved in a cell signaling pathway. The interaction between different cell types promotes full harmony of their various and vital functions: regulation, homeostasis, immune response, and protection of the host integrity. The alteration of any of these functions causes serious pathological disorders, including autoimmune diseases, cancers, immune deficiencies, and allergic diseases. Finally, a healthy immune system could be described by five main features: (i) self- and non–self-recognition, (ii) non–self-rejection, (iii) modified-self rejection, (iv) tolerance of unmodified self-components, and (v) coherence and integrity.

can also recognize and bind substances released from damaged host tissues and cells (damage-associated molecular patterns, DAMPs) [4].

The cells of the adaptive immune system—B cells and T cells—are derived from the same pluripotent hematopoietic stem cells [5]. These cells carry on their surface highly diversified antigen-specific receptors, which are able of interacting with a quasi-unlimited number of antigens, thanks to their structure diversity. B cells specifically recognize and bind intact antigens, through highly variable domains of their cell-surface receptors (B cell receptors, BCR), whereas T cells specifically recognize and interact via the highly variable domains of their receptors (T cell receptors, TCR) with peptide fragments derived from antigens in association with major histocompatibility complex (MHC) molecules on the surface of antigen-presenting cells (APCs) [6]. Two classes of such cells have been defined by their functions and their differentiation markers (cluster of differentiation, CD), but also by the class of MHC molecules they recognize: $CD4^+$ helper T cells and $CD8^+$ cytotoxic T cells that interact with peptide-class-II-MHC and peptide-class-I-MHC complexes, respectively [5]. The subset of $CD4^+$ T cells that express high levels of CD25 ($CD4^+$ $CD25^{high}$), so-called regulatory T cells (Tregs), is essential in maintaining immunological self-tolerance and prevention of autoimmunity. A deleterious autoimmune reaction may be generated as a result of decreased frequency and/or function of Treg cells in both organ-specific and systemic autoimmune diseases [7]. Of note, regulatory cells are not limited to $CD4^+$ T cells but can include various immune cell subsets, such as $CD8^+$ Treg, Tr1 regulatory cells, Th3 cells, natural killer like T (NKT) cells, and Breg cells [8–10] that can prevent destructive immune responses and autoimmunity. Additionally, to establish a self-tolerance by the immune system, potentially dangerous autoreactive T cell and B cell clones must be deleted through negative selection or clonal deletion within mechanisms of central tolerance occurred in the thymus and bone marrow, respectively, before they develop into fully immunocompetent cells [11, 12]. Failure or breakdown of negative selection, which can also occur in the periphery, can lead to the development of autoimmunity and autoimmune diseases [11–15].

3. Reactions against self-antigens and autoimmunity

When the immune system is abnormally overactivated, as a result of defective regulation function, and triggers a strong reaction against its unmodified components, autoimmune pathological manifestations might develop. Autoimmune responses involve, as a classical immune response, T cells, B cells, APCs, inflammatory cells, antibodies, and many other mediators of immunity such as cytokines.

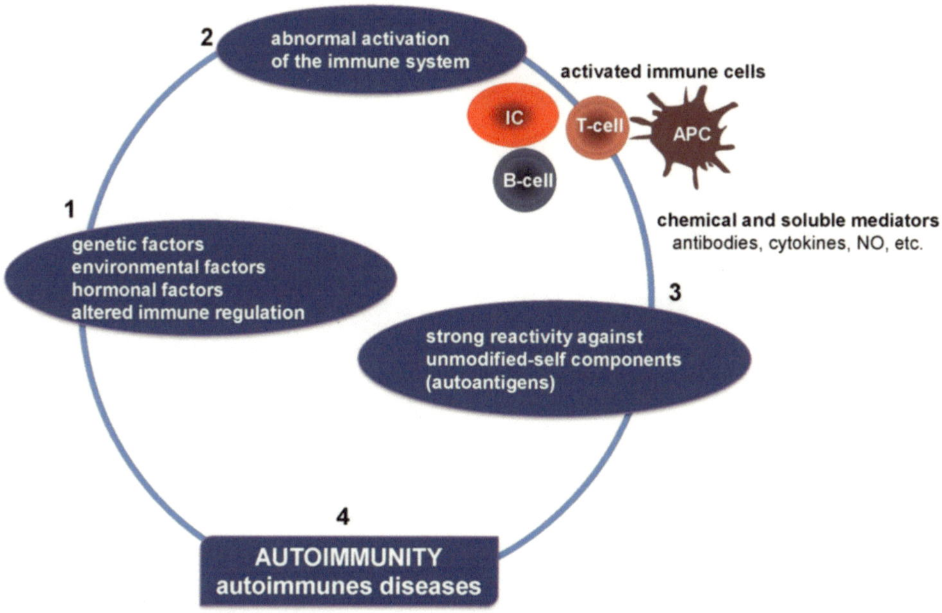

Figure 2. Pathophysiological mechanisms of autoimmune diseases. Autoimmune diseases are multifactorial diseases, and their etiologies are not yet fully known. Their development depends on genetic susceptibility, environmental factors, hormonal factors, and immune dysregulation. These factors may influence, according to different mechanisms, the abnormal activation of potentially dangerous autoreactive cells. Other components are involved in enhancing the autoimmune process, including, antigen-presenting cells, inflammatory cells, and many chemical and soluble mediators such as vasoactive amines, nitric oxide, lipid mediators, growth factors, complement system, cytokines, etc. APC, antigen-presenting cell; IC, inflammatory cell; NO, nitric oxide.

Numerous factors have been associated to pathological autoimmunity, including genetic predisposition and epigenetic change, environmental factors (nutrition, viral and bacterial infection, and ultraviolet radiation), drugs (beta-blockers, antipsychotics, and antibiotics), vaccination, sex hormone, etc. [16–22] (**Figure 2**).

4. Autoimmune diseases

Autoimmune diseases and autoimmune-related diseases are numerous (there are more than 130, AARDA). Some of them are more severe or more frequent than others. They are conventionally distinguished in organ-specific autoimmune diseases, in which the autoantigen target is localized in one organ or tissue, and systemic or nonorgan specific autoimmune diseases in which autoantigens are widely distributed in the body or spread throughout several organs (**Figure 3**). In addition, common autoimmune disorders can coexist in the same patient [27, 28], which further complicates diagnosis and medical management.

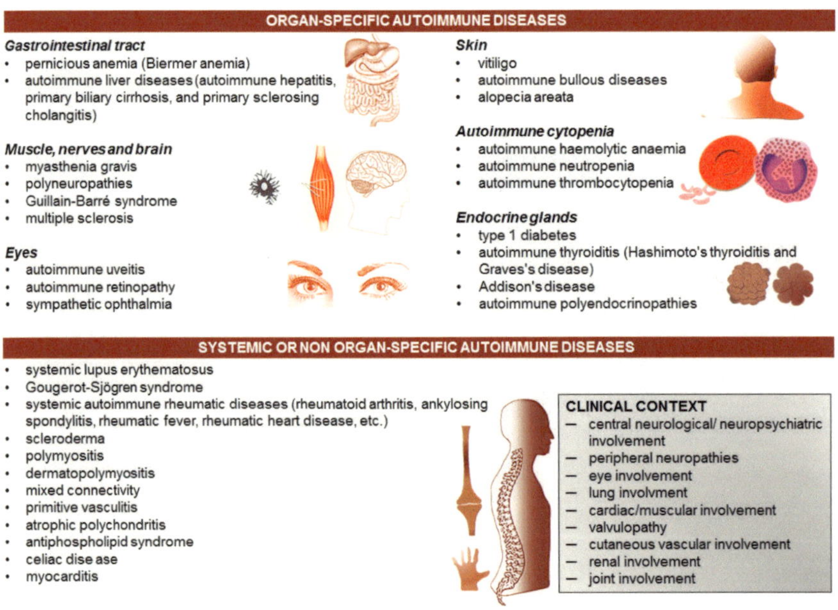

Figure 3. Types of autoimmune diseases. There are two categories of autoimmune diseases: organ-specific autoimmune diseases and nonorgan specific autoimmune diseases, also called systemic diseases. Organ-specific autoimmune diseases are restricted to certain organs or a particular tissue. Nonorgan specific autoimmune diseases are characterized by extensive lesions that are secondary to an autoimmune reaction against ubiquitous autoantigens. There are also many overlap syndromes that may be characterized by the association of two or more organ-specific and systemic autoimmune diseases, due probably to the existence of common immunogenetic factors. Finally, such categorization of autoimmune diseases does not take into account diseases resulting from immune reactions against foreign antigens expressed in a target tissue, especially in viral diseases. It also ignores autoimmunity observed under physiological conditions in the absence of any pathological tissue damage [23–26]. (The list of pathologies presented in this figure is not exhaustive.).

http://dx.doi.org/10.5772/67671

Although it is not easy to determine for each individual the exact cause of pathological autoimmunity, given the extensive heterogeneity of autoimmune disorders [29], relevant research strategies with advanced technologies are developed or are still under investigation to control or prevent these diseases in a wider context (**Figure 4**).

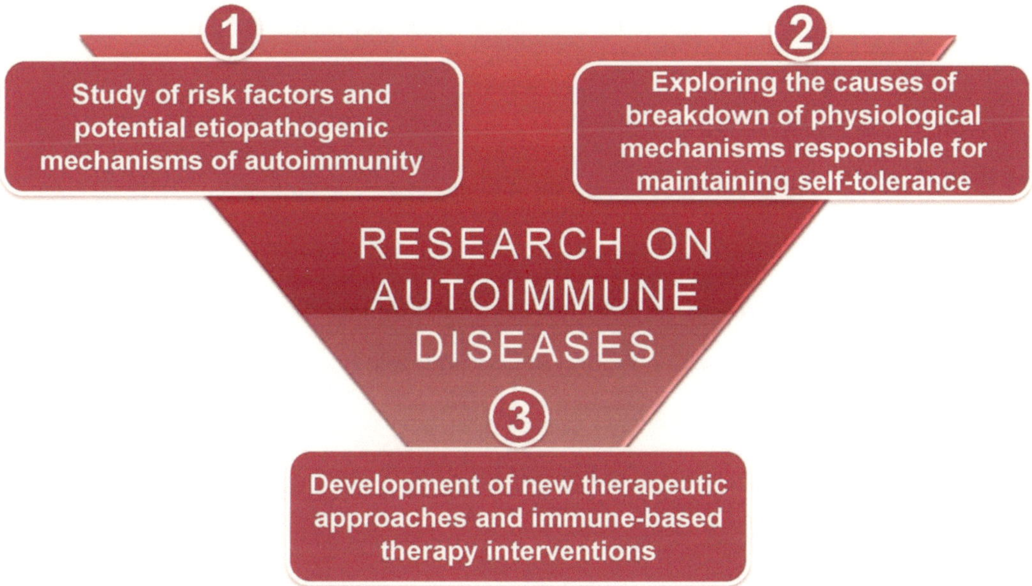

Figure 4. Strategies for exploring autoimmune diseases. The exact causes of autoimmune diseases are not yet fully understood, but are the subject of intensive researches that are focused mainly on three main axes: (i) study of the risk factors and potential etiopathogenetic mechanisms underlying these illnesses, (ii) research on the causes of the breakdown of the mechanisms responsible for maintaining tolerance to self-antigens, and (iii) development of innovative therapies and immune interventions. Current treatments aim to suppress autoimmune response and inflammation and alleviate the functional consequences of cellular or tissue damage.

5. Conclusions

The essential function of the immune system is the eradication of aggressive elements, particularly infectious agents and tumor cells. In order to ensure normal immune functions, lymphocyte clones which are capable of strongly recognizing harmless or unmodified elements of the self are eliminated or suppressed so that under normal conditions no autoimmune reaction is observed.

The explosion of knowledge thanks to molecular biology over the past few decades has opened new perspectives in the search for risk factors that could be directly involved in the occurrence of autoimmune diseases. It is now well-established that these diseases may be caused by a combination of a genetic predisposition and a triggering factor.

More than 130 autoimmune diseases and autoimmune-related diseases have been identified. Most often, a distinction is made between organ-specific autoimmune diseases, for which specific organs are the target of an attack by the immune system, and nonorgan specific autoimmune diseases which are of a systemic manifestation.

Significant progress has been made in understanding the etiopathogenetic mechanisms of autoimmune diseases. They should undoubtedly lead to more effective therapeutic strategies. Currently, there are multiple potential treatments that often rely on immunosuppression. Nevertheless, the best strategy would be to act more selectively on the self-reactive cells that are abnormally overactives.

Author details

Mourad Aribi

*Address all correspondence to: m_aribi@mail.univ-tlemcen.dz

Laboratory of Applied Molecular Biology and Immunology, Tlemcen Abou-Bekr Belkaïd University, Tlemcen, Algeria

References

[1] Dembic Z. Immune system protects integrity of tissues. Mol Immunol 2000;37:563–9.

[2] Dembic Z. Response to Cohn: The immune system rejects the harmful, protects the useful and neglects the rest of microorganisms. Scand J Immunol 2004;60:3–5. doi:10.1111/j.0300-9475.2004.01451.x.

[3] Revillard J-P, Association of Immunology Teachers of French-language Universities. Immunology. Paris: De Boeck & Larcier; 2001.

[4] Portnoy JM, Williams PB, Barnes CS. Innate immune responses to fungal allergens. Curr Allergy Asthma Rep 2016;16:62. doi:10.1007/s11882-016-0643-4.

[5] Janeway CA, editor. Immunobiology: The immune system in health and disease [animated CD-ROM inside]. 5th ed. New York, NY: Garland Publisher; 2001.

[6] Andersen PS, Stryhn A, Hansen BE, Fugger L, Engberg J, Buus S. A recombinant antibody with the antigen-specific, major histocompatibility complex-restricted specificity of T cells. Proc Natl Acad Sci USA 1996;93:1820–4.

[7] Valencia X, Lipsky PE. CD4+CD25+FoxP3+ regulatory T cells in autoimmune diseases. Nat Clin Pract Rheumatol 2007;3:619–26. doi:10.1038/ncprheum0624.

[8] Azizi G, Pouyani MR, Abolhassani H, Sharifi L, Dizaji MZ, Mohammadi J, et al. Cellular and molecular mechanisms of immune dysregulation and autoimmunity. Cell Immunol 2016;310:14–26. doi:10.1016/j.cellimm.2016.08.012.

[9] Gol-Ara M, Jadidi-Niaragh F, Sadria R, Azizi G, Mirshafiey A. The role of different subsets of regulatory T cells in immunopathogenesis of rheumatoid arthritis. Arthritis 2012;2012:805875. doi:10.1155/2012/805875.

[10] Yang M, Rui K, Wang S, Lu L. Regulatory B cells in autoimmune diseases. Cell Mol Immunol 2013;10:122–32. doi:10.1038/cmi.2012.60.

[11] Anderton SM, Wraith DC. Selection and fine-tuning of the autoimmune T-cell repertoire. Nat Rev Immunol 2002;2:487–98. doi:10.1038/nri842.

[12] Sandel PC, Monroe JG. Negative selection of immature B cells by receptor editing or deletion is determined by site of antigen encounter. Immunity 1999;10:289–99.

[13] Romagnani S. Immunological tolerance and autoimmunity. Intern Emerg Med 2006;1: 187–96.

[14] Strasser A, Puthalakath H, O'Reilly LA, Bouillet P. What do we know about the mechanisms of elimination of autoreactive T and B cells and what challenges remain. Immunol Cell Biol 2008;86:57–66. doi:10.1038/sj.icb.7100141.

[15] Giltiay NV, Lu Y, Allman D, Jørgensen TN, Li X. The adaptor molecule Act1 regulates BAFF responsiveness and self-reactive B cell selection during transitional B cell maturation. J Immunol 2010;185:99–109. doi:10.4049/jimmunol.0903312.

[16] Hewagama A, Richardson B. The genetics and epigenetics of autoimmune diseases. J Autoimmun 2009;33:3–11. doi:10.1016/j.jaut.2009.03.007.

[17] Takorabet L, Ropars A, Raby C, Charreire J. Phenothiazine induces de novo MHC class II antigen expression on thyroid epithelial cells. A new mechanism for drug-induced autoimmunity. J Immunol 1995;154:3593–602.

[18] Steel NR, Taylor JJ, Young ET, Farndon JR, Holcombe M, Kendall-Taylor P. The effect of subtotal thyroidectomy with propranolol preparation on antibody activity in Graves' disease. Clin Endocrinol (Oxf) 1987;26:97–106.

[19] Rosser EC, Mauri C. A clinical update on the significance of the gut microbiota in systemic autoimmunity. J Autoimmun 2016;74:85–93. doi:10.1016/j.jaut.2016.06.009.

[20] Silvester JA, Leffler DA. Is autoimmunity infectious? The effect of gastrointestinal viral infections and vaccination on risk of celiac disease autoimmunity. Clin Gastroenterol Hepatol Off Clin Pract J Am Gastroenterol Assoc 2016. doi:10.1016/j.cgh.2016.12.014.

[21] Dahan S, Shoenfeld Y. Letter to the editor—HPV vaccine and autoimmunity incidence of new-onset autoimmune disease in girls and women with pre-existing autoimmune disease after quadrivalent human papillomavirus vaccination: a cohort study. J Intern Med 2016. doi:10.1111/joim.12575.

[22] Karaca Z, Laway BA, Dokmetas HS, Atmaca H, Kelestimur F. Sheehan syndrome. Nat Rev Dis Primer 2016;2:16092. doi:10.1038/nrdp.2016.92.

[23] Bach J-F, Chatenoud L. Immunologie. Paris: Médecine-Sciences Flammarion;2002.

[24] Owlia MB, Mostafavi Pour Manshadi SMY, Naderi N. Cardiac manifestations of rheumatological conditions: A narrative review. ISRN Rheumatol 2012;2012:463620. doi:10.5402/2012/463620.

[25] Elebute M, Marsh J. Autoimmune cytopenias. Medicine (Baltimore) 2009;37:159–63. doi:10.1016/j.mpmed.2008.12.008.

[26] Washington MK. Autoimmune liver disease: Overlap and outliers. Mod Pathol Off J U S Can Acad Pathol Inc 2007;20 Suppl 1:S15–30. doi:10.1038/modpathol.3800684.

[27] Fridkis-Hareli M. Immunogenetic mechanisms for the coexistence of organ-specific and systemic autoimmune diseases. J Autoimmune Dis 2008;5:1. doi:10.1186/1740-2557-5-1.

[28] Boelaert K, Newby PR, Simmonds MJ, Holder RL, Carr-Smith JD, Heward JM, et al. Prevalence and relative risk of other autoimmune diseases in subjects with autoimmune thyroid disease. Am J Med 2010;123:183.e1–9. doi:10.1016/j.amjmed.2009.06.030.

[29] Cho JH, Feldman M. Heterogeneity of autoimmune diseases: pathophysiologic insights from genetics and implications for new therapies. Nat Med 2015;21:730–8.doi:10.1038/nm.3897.

Chapter 2

Immunotherapy in Autoimmune Diabetes

Mohammad Haque, Praneet Sandhu, Swetha Ravi,

Sravya Kurapati and Jianxun Song

Additional information is available at the end of the chapter

http://dx.doi.org/10.5772/66909

Abstract

Autoimmune diabetes is a chronic autoimmune disease caused by the loss or selective destruction of the insulin-producing cells, called pancreatic beta cells. Damage to beta cells results in an absence or insufficient production of insulin produced by the body. Most cases of autoimmune diabetes have an autoimmune basis, and the immune system mistakenly attacks and destroys beta cells. The immune system plays a critical role in controlling the development of autoimmune diabetes. Over the past years there have been significant progress and an accumulation of scientific evidence for the concept of immunotherapy. Immunotherapy for the prevention and treatment of autoimmune diabetes has become the main focus of the research community. Three regimens of immunotherapy have been investigated: (1) Antigen-specific vaccines: Insulin-related molecules have attracted great interest in vaccine development, including the whole recombinant human GAD65 (rhGAD65) and the DiaPep277 peptide of HSP60. (2) Systemic immunomodulators: A large number of non–antigen-specific immunomodulators have been studied, including monoclonal anti-CD3 antibody, anti–CTLA-4 Ig, TNF-a, IFN-a, IL-1R antagonist, regulatory T cells, and dendritic cells. (3) Combination treatments: Combination therapies have the ability to enhance efficacy and will become the standard of care for autoimmune diabetes. Development of safe and efficient prevention of autoimmune diabetes is a general public health object in modern countries now. Although large numbers of preventive modalities including immunotherapy have been accomplished in animal models of autoimmune diabetes, prevention of human autoimmune diabetes remains indefinable. Genetic and environmental factors that control the relapsing-remitting course of β-cell destruction, terminating in complete insulin addiction are being determined. In the long run, initial prevention of islet autoimmunity will likely be the optimal approach to the prevention of autoimmune diabetes. However, environmental causes of islet autoimmunity need to be well stated. Modest predictive assessment of the existing genetic screening tools also means that the number of children requiring intervention will stay great, concerning the number of autoimmune diabetes cases prohibited. Nevertheless, combination treatments are more likely to be used for autoimmune diabetes. Primary systemic immunosuppression followed by antigen-specific induction of tolerance or islet regeneration is a sound approach.

Keywords: autoimmune diabetes, immunotherapy, immune cells, tolerance

1. Introduction

Autoimmune diseases arise due to loss of self-tolerance caused by tissue injury by T cells or antibody reactivity to self. There are several causes of autoimmunity that are not fully understood. One of the major causes of autoimmune disease is the activation of self-reactive T and B lymphocytes. During T and B cell development, Self-reactive T and B cells should be eliminated by antigen ligation of T cell receptor or B cell receptor. This is known as the mechanism of self-tolerance. To maintain the self-tolerance and eliminate the autoreactive cell, T cells and B cells undergo a selection process in primary lymphoid organs, the thymus and the bone marrow, respectively [1–3]. After somatic mutation of immunoglobulin genes, B cells need to go through a second process of selection failing which somatic mutation generates auto reactivity. This is called central tolerance. If somehow, central tolerance is not maintained, autoimmunity develops. Several autoimmune diseases have been reported until now. Among them, type-1 diabetes (T1D) is one of the major autoimmune diseases that develop due to the selective autoimmune destruction of pancreatic beta cells that leads to the insulin insufficiency. There is no definite treatment for T1D except life-long insulin therapy. Hence, the generation of insulin secreting beta cells and transplanting it to the diabetic patients is an unmet need.

Pluripotent stem cells (PSCs) have the ability to grow indefinitely while maintaining pluripotency. Under the right circumstances, mouse and human stem cells have the potential ability to differentiate into disease-relevant cells [4]. The generation of exogenous beta cells and its transplantation to replace dead or dysfunctional endogenous beta cell is a potential strategy for controlling blood glucose level in diabetic patients. Stem cell-derived beta cells have already been generated previously, and it was successfully able to control the blood glucose in clinical settings [5]. As autoimmune disease is a continuous process, it is possible to develop diabetes again by destructing the pancreatic islets by pathogenic T cells. As a result, this will not be a permanent solution for the control of blood glucose level.

It is already well established that regulatory T cells (Tregs), one of the subtype of T cells, are able to suppress the hyper activity of other T cells including beta cell-destructing pathogenic T cells. But the number of Tregs is relatively limited in mice and human being. The generation of Tregs *in vitro* and adoptively transfer them into the diabetic mice will be a great strategy for the treatment of diabetes that will reduce the hazards of complicated surgery events throughout the life. We already showed that retroviral transduction of genes with T cell receptor (TCR) and the transcriptional factor (FoxP3) into PSCs following coculture with stromal OP9-DL1/DL4 cells differentiate them into antigen (Ag)-specific Tregs. Our *in vitro* generated Tregs were able to suppress the autoimmune arthritis in a well-established mouse model of Ag-induced arthritis (AIA) [6, 7]. In this chapter, we will discuss how Ag-specific

Tregs can be generated from PSCs and how they are able to reduce blood glucose level in a mouse model of diabetes.

1.1. Epidemiology: incidence and prevalence

T1D is one of the most common chronic diseases in children. Children under 18 years of age are mostly affected. In 2012, 29.1 million Americans, or 9.3% of the population, had diabetes. More than 150,000 children in the United States have T1D; 1.4 million Americans are diagnosed with diabetes each year [8]. In children, T1D develops between 5 and 7 years of age and at puberty. The incidence for the development of T1D also varies with seasonal changes and geography. It seems that autumn and winter are the seasons for higher incidence of diabetes as compared to summer. The incidence and prevalence dramatically vary around the world, where some countries have 400-fold higher incidence rate compared to the others. The incidence rates of diabetes in China, India, and Venezuela are 0.1 per 100,000 and are far more common in Finland. In Finland, the incidence is approaching 50 cases per 100,000 individuals per year. Wide variations have been observed between neighboring areas in Europe and North America. Estonia is very close to Finland but the incidence of diabetes is less than one-third as that of Finland. Puerto Rico has an incidence similar to that of the mainland United States, whereas neighboring Cuba has an incidence of less than 3 cases per 100,000 [9].

The incidence for the development of T1D is increasing throughout the world. These changes are markedly observed in young children from countries with historically high incidence rates. Sweden and Norway have reported 3.3% annual increase in T1D rates, and Finland has observed a 2.4% annual rise in incidence. Hence, the increase in T1D incidence is not correlated with socio-economic condition. Most of the autoimmune diseases disproportionally affect women but T1D seems to affect men and women equally. Therefore, T1D is different in disease prevalence and incidence that suggests that it is a combination of multiple genetic and environmental factors.

1.2. Etiology

T1D is the result of an autoimmune reaction to the proteins of pancreatic islets. There is a strong association between T1D and other autoimmune diseases such as Addison's disease. It is also notable that the incidence of autoimmune diseases is increased in family members of T1D patients. T1D develops due to the destruction of pancreatic beta cells by autoreactive T cells. Other types of diabetes may also develop due to a combination of reduced insulin sensitivity and impaired beta cells function [10]. Diabetes can be inherited or caused by mutations in an autosomal dominant gene resulting in the disruption of insulin production. There are three types of autoantibodies that are involved in the development of T1D:

1. Islet cell cytoplasmic antibodies: the presence of islet cell cytoplasmic antibodies indicates the future development of diabetes. Note that 90% of T1D antibodies are against islet cell cytoplasmic protein.

2. Islet cell surface antibodies: there are some other antibodies that are directed toward the islet cell surface Ags. Autoantibody against islet cell surface Ag is also detected in almost 80% of the cases. These antibodies are also positive in type 2 diabetes.

3. Specific antigenic target of islet cell: 80% newly diagnosed patients represent with autoantibody to glutamic acid decarboxylase (GAD). Presence of this antibody is also a strong predictor for future development of T1D. Anti-GAD antibody declines over time in T1D. In some cases, anti-insulin antibodies are also detected in T1D patients and in relatives [11].

In some cases, some viruses like B4 strain of the coxsackie B virus, German measles, Mumps, and Rota viruses are also responsible for the development of diabetes. When a virus invades the body, T cells start to produce antibodies against that virus. If some viruses have the same Ag as the beta cells, T cells can actually turn against the beta cell and start destroying it.

There is a strong genetic correlation for the development of diabetes though it is not an inheritance. It is considered as a complex and multifactorial disease. In the United States, individuals who have first-degree relative with T1D have 5% risk for the development of diabetes. But in general population this percentage is very low. Monozygotic twins have a high risk whereas dizygotic twins have a lower risk. There are a significant percentage of people developing diabetes without any family history. Differences in risk are also developed in the parents of children. Children who have their mother suffering from T1D have 2% risk of developing T1D, but children whose fathers have diabetes have a greater risk [12]. No single gene is predicted to develop diabetes, but more than two dozen susceptibility loci have been associated with susceptibility to T1D.

2. Pathophysiologic mechanism of T1D

The main factor for the development of autoimmune diabetes is loss of immunologic tolerance to β cells. β cells are selectively destructed by autoimmune reaction. Due to loss of immunologic tolerance, autoreactive $CD4^+$ and $CD8^+$ T cells as well as macrophages are infiltrated into the pancreatic islet and develop insulitis. During the disease process, several autoantigen that are targeted by autoantibodies are detected into the islet. The main autoantigen that may be found in the islets are insulin, glutamic acid decarboxylase (GAD65), islet Ag-2 (IA-2), and zinc transporter (ZnT8). These autoantibodies are predominantly associated with the development of insulitis [13]. Destruction of β cells is not dependent only on autoantigen, it is also related to the presence of high-risk human leukocyte antigen (HLA) haplotypes like DR3-DQ2, DR4-DQ8, or both [14]. HLA-class II molecules are mainly expressed by Ag-presenting cells (APC) like dendritic cells (DCs) and macrophage. In some cases, they are expressed by activated $CD4^+$ and B cells, even on activated endothelial cells. The presence of high-risk HLA molecules on APC may activate $CD8^+$ T cells through $CD4^+$ T lymphocytes. Then $CD8^+$ T cells become hyperactivated and initiate the destruction of β cells. This phenomenon is implicated in T1D siblings who share the high-risk HLA DR3-DQ2/DR4-DQ8 genotype [15].

Some other pathophysiological mechanisms have been documented. But the two most common mechanisms for developing T1D are:

1. Gradual β-cell destruction associated with one or multiple islet cell autoantibodies.

2. Development of glucose intolerance and hyperglycemia due to loss of β-cell secretory function.

The autoimmune process starts with the infiltration of mononuclear cells including autoreactive $CD8^+$ T cells into the pancreas that leads to the destruction of β cell. In the disease process, both the cellular and humoral pathways of immunity are involved. However, the role of B lymphocytes is not evident in human, only in the laboratory animal such as nonobese diabetic (NOD) mice [5]. In NOD mice, B cells infiltrate in the islets of young mice and play a role in the initiation of β-cell destruction by the autoimmune response. In some other autoimmune diseases like rheumatoid arthritis, systemic lupus erythematosus, and multiple sclerosis B-cell-targeted therapy has been used successfully.

There are several features that characterize the T1D as an autoimmune disease. These are because of the presence of mononuclear and immunocompetent cells in the infiltrated pancreatic islets; association with the class II major histocompatibility complex; islets cell-specific auto-antibodies; increase in the number of $CD8^+$ T cells in the pancreas and reduction in the number of $CD4^+$ T cell; and response to immunotherapy and other organ-specific autoimmune diseases.

The hallmark of T1D is the selective destruction of pancreatic islets. But due to marked heterogeneity, it is difficult to follow the destruction of beta cells within the islets. At the onset of hyperglycemia islet contain numerous components like infiltrating lymphocytes and monocytes, a mixture of pseudo-atrophic islets, pancreatic polypeptide, and somatostatin [16]. Lymphocyte infiltration is prominent when diabetes becomes chronic. Another important prerequisite for the development of diabetes is the activation of islet Ag-specific $CD4^+$ T cell [17]. Transferring of $CD4^+$ T cells into the nondiabetic mice from diabetic mice also developed insulitis and diabetes. It is already reported that $CD4^+$ T cells are able to induce diabetes initially and $CD8^+$ T cells participate in damaging the pancreas [18]. Some cytokines are also responsible for the development of autoimmune diabetes. High level of IL-2 and IFN-α correlates or enhances the induction of autoimmune diabetes by activating the macrophage in experimental models [19]. In the process of infiltration, macrophages are the first cell type invading the islets where they produce TNF-alpha and IL-1. TNF-alpha and IL-1 play an important role for inducing the structural changes of beta cells and suppression of their insulin releasing capacity.

3. T1D and Tregs

The role of Tregs has been focused in various autoimmune diseases. The vast majority of $CD4^+$ and $CD8^+$ T cells are eliminated in the thymus through central tolerance induction mechanism. But in some cases, few autoreactive T cells are not eliminated and are released to the peripheral circulation. These autoreactive T cells migrate into the pancreas that causes the destruction of islets cells and develop diabetes if they are not actively suppressed by Tregs. T1D is mainly a T cell-mediated autoimmune disease where pancreatic beta cells are destroyed due to the breakdown of tolerance to islets Ag. Initially, autoreactive $CD4^+$ T cell subset recognizes self-Ag and produce T helper (Th) 1 cytokine spectrum that initiate the autoimmune process. For further processing, $CD8^+$ T cells are necessary [20]. Tregs have the ability to prevent self-reactivity through active suppression [21]. Several studies have demonstrated that $CD4^+$ $CD25^+$ Tregs expressing FoxP3 play an indispensable role in the maintenance of immune homeostasis by regulating inflammatory response against invading pathogens and preventing destruction of autoimmunity [22, 23].

There are a number of autoantigens that are involved in the pathogenesis of T1D. But the true primary autoantigen in T1D has not yet been definitively identified. It is very important to identify the islet-specific autoantigen for the development of autoantigen-specific tolerance induction immunotherapy and for establishing diagnostic and predictive markers of T1D. Until now, the most accepted autoimmune features of T1D are the presence of autoreactive T cells and autoantibodies in the pancreas. It is also proposed that autoantibody against islet autoantigen may appear many years before clinical diagnosis; 90% patients with T1D exhibit autoantibodies against islets autoantigen. But it is not clear whether these autoantibodies play a pathogenic role for the development of diabetes. Studies of different animal and human models lacking with certain types of cells demonstrated that the lack of Tregs or impairment of their function lead to the development of autoimmune disease, including diabetes [24, 25].

A number of mouse models suggests that Tregs play an important role to prevent the onset of diabetes. But how the Tregs can function *in vivo* to block the development of diabetes are still under investigation. There are some mechanisms that were proposed on the basis of mouse models, and its clinical significance is yet to be proved. As autoreactive T cells are the main culprits for the development of diabetes, it is essential to control the migration or differentiation of autoreactive T cells into the pancreatic lymph node. Tregs present in the pancreatic lymph node have the ability to regulate the priming of autoreactive T cells by limiting their expansion and differentiation. Tregs also have the ability to interrupt the development of autoreactive T cells through limiting the access of autoreactive T cells to DCs [26]. By limiting the priming of T cells in the lymph nodes, Treg cell also prevent the T cells becoming an effector T cells. Infiltration of autoreactive T cells into the islet is a crucial step for the development of inflammation and leading to the destruction of islet. Some chemokine receptors like chemokine receptor 3 (CXCR3) secreted by effector T cells are essential for infiltrating them into the islets. By exerting their suppressing mechanism, Tregs inhibit the expression of CXCR3 and ultimately prevents the infiltration of these cells into the pancreatic islets. The most common suppressive cytokine IL-10 and TGF-beta are secreted by inducible Tregs [27, 28]. These two cytokines play an important immunoregulatory role in T1D. TGF-beta secreted by Tregs in the islet during the priming phase stimulates the expansion or generation of intra-islet FoxP3 expressing Tregs [29]. It is already established that increased numbers of Tregs are essential for the suppression of autoreactive T cells that are destructive to the islets. Migration of autoreactive T cells into the islet worsens the disease condition. Intracellular adhesion molecule 1 (ICAM1) is one of the potential factors that helps to migrate the autoreactive T cells into the islets. ICAM1 is exclusively expressed by autoreactive $CD4^+$ and $CD8^+$ T cells [30, 31]. IL-10 secreted by Tregs downregulates the expression of ICAM1 on effector T cells, which prevents their migration to the target organ [32]. IL-10 also reduces the hyperactivity of T cells by modulating the function of APC and reduces the inflammation [33].

4. Role of Tregs in autoimmunity

Tregs are a subset of T cells that exhibit inhibitory or regulatory effects on effector T cells. Previously it was known as suppressor T cells. There is a phenotypical variation of Tregs, such as $CD4^{+}CD25^{+}FoxP3^{+}$ Tregs, $CD8^{+}$ Tregs, and $CD3^{+}$ $CD4^{-}CD8^{-}$ Tregs [34, 35]. A dysfunction, defect, or absence of Tregs has been implicated in the pathogenesis of many autoimmune diseases [36] as they are indispensable to maintain the immune homeostasis. However, how they control the development of autoimmunity is still under debate. Previous data suggests that several numbers of genetic and mechanistic defects may arise leading to defective regulation by Tregs [37]. Though all different types of Tregs work together to maintain the homeostasis, $CD4^{+}$ $FoxP3^{+}$ Tregs play the major role because they are the long lasting and produce most of the suppressive cytokines. There are several mechanisms by which Tregs exert their regulatory effects on effector T cells. These are cell-to-cell contact, secretion of IL-10 and TGF-beta-like immunosuppressive cytokines, modification or killing of APC, and competition for growth factor [38, 39]. $CD4^{+}$ $FoxP3^{+}$ Tregs suppresses the immune response, inflammation, and tissue destruction by inhibiting the function of classical $CD4^{+}$ Th cells, antibody production of B cells, and $CD8^{+}$ cytotoxic T lymphocyte granule release. Inducible $CD4^{+}$ $foxP3^{-}$ type 1 Tregs or $CD4^{+}FoxP3^{+}$ Tregs can exhibit their suppressive function through IL-10 secretion. Though some other functions of Tregs have been documented but the major function is to maintain the immune homeostasis. Deficiency in Treg frequency or function results in imbalance in the immune system. But in some cases there are no apparent defects in Treg frequencies like multiple sclerosis [40]. The result in other autoimmune settings have been mixed, but overall in most autoimmune patients, ample number of Tregs appear in the circulation. Any discrepancies in the results reflects the nonspecific phenotypic markers available or due to contamination with non-Tregs. Until now, almost all studies have been limited to analysis of peripheral blood so it is difficult to understand what is happening at the site of inflammation. A number of studies showed reduced frequencies of Tregs in peripheral blood, but an increased number or potency of cells isolated from inflammatory sites [41]. This may be a compensatory mechanism in response to ongoing inflammation during the disease process. Treg stability is another important issue when assessing the frequency of Tregs. Many autoimmune diseases are thought to undergo periods of relapse and remission [42]. These variations are susceptible to the influence of immunosuppressive regimens used in the treatment of autoimmune disease. Moreover, during the progression of disease Tregs in local sites can change phenotypically.

5. Management of T1D

T1D is a chronic metabolic disorder characterized by deficiency of insulin production by pancreatic beta cells. Insulin is essential for maintaining the normal blood glucose level. As it is an autoimmune destruction caused by endogenous autoreactive T cells, exogenous insulin supply is required to maintain normoglycemia in many diabetic patients. This is a lifelong treatment that is not convenient. Another option for treatment is replacement of beta cell therapy where sufficient amount of beta cells need to be included to control the blood glucose level without repeated insulin injection. However, the beta cell transplantation did not achieve a satisfactory result. In 2000, Shapiro and colleagues achieved independence of insulin injections in seven T1D patients by transplanting a large number of islet cells combined with the use of glucocorticoid-free immunosuppressive regimen [43]. But the insulin independency was not sustained for long. Some patients even had complete graft loss 1 year after the final transplantation. The main reason for poor long-term outcome is continuous immune destruction of the transplanted islet as autoimmune destruction is a continuous process. Beta cell transplantation also has a major obstacle, shortage of donors when compared with large population. As cadaver tissue provides a low yield of islet cells, it requires a large number of donor cells to generate sufficient insulin-producing beta cells that are capable of producing and releasing adequate amount of insulin in response to normal physiological signals. Furthermore, chronic immunosuppression is also necessary after allograft transplantation. Patient-specific islet-like cells from adult tissues may compensate both the shortage of organ donors and allograft rejection. Several groups were successful to generate functional islet-like clusters from adult progenitor cells, but their success were limited [44, 45]. Therefore, it is highly demanding to explore some other option for searching more defined sources of beta cells.

Generation of induced PSCs (iPSCs) opens a new era in the treatment of autoimmune diseases. IPSCs have the ability to become all kinds of cells if they are maintained properly [46]. As Tregs have the ability to Suppress the hyper activity of autoreactive T cells and they can be expanded *in vivo* after one-time transplant, it is ideal to generate Tregs from iPSCs for the treatment of autoimmune diabetes.

6. iPSCs

Due to restricted use of human embryonic stem cells (ESCs) in both research and clinical settings, induced pluripotent stem cells (iPSCs) serve as an attractive potential alternative to ESCs. Human somatic cells can be reverted back to pluripotent stem cells by expression of defined transcription factors. Mouse and human somatic cells have already been converted into iPSCs by introducing transcription factors OCT4, and SOX2 in combination with KLF4, c-MYC, NANOG, and lin-28 homolog A [47]. iPSCs are similar to ESCs in morphology, gene expression, epigenetic status, and *in vitro* differentiation. C-MYC and KLF4 are known oncogenes and their use to generate iPSCs raises concerns about potential tumor formation. However, this can be overcome by the use of a histone deacytylase inhibitor, valproic acid, which facilitates the reprogramming of primary human fibroblasts with only two factors, OCT4 and SOX2. Thus, the reprogramming of cells to pluripotency has become potentially safer and practical for therapeutic use [48]. Another challenge was the use of retrovirus or lentivirus to deliver transcription factor genes into the somatic cells. This also raised the concern about viral integration into the host genome that increases risk of tumorigenicity. To avoid this risk, Yamanaka used a novel repeated transfection protocol for the expression of plasmids that resulted in iPSCs without evidence of plasmid integration [49]. Other groups also generated iPSCs from umbilical cord blood by lentiviral overexpression of the reprogramming factor OCT4, SOX2, NANOG, and LIN28 [50]. The reprogramming efficiency was almost the same as keratinocytes and fibroblast. However, use of umbilical cord blood also leads to a possibility that it may be mutated over the lifetime of an organism. Thus, it is still under debate whether iPSCs are truly equivalent to human ESCs or not with respect to pluripotency.

iPSCs have already been used for the generation of Insulin secreting cells. iPSCs were generated from skin biopsies of a patient with T1D by using three transcription factors OCT4, SOX2, and KLF4 [51]. These cells were differentiated into insulin-producing cells. These cells were found to be released human C-peptide and exhibited a five-fold increase in the secretion of C-peptide in response to 20 mM glucose, which reveals that functional beta cells can eventually be derived from iPSCs.

Generation of functional beta cells for the immunotherapy of T1D is not the only challenge; there is a need to overcome the immune response both in terms of autoimmunity and rejection of allogenic tissue. It is also unknown whether these *in vitro* generated cells will migrate to the target tissue or not. Since beta cells will continuously be destroyed upon development of autoimmunity, it is ideal to generate Ag or tissue-specific Tregs from iPSCs for the treatments of autoimmune diabetes.

7. Generation of Ag/tissue-specific Tregs from iPSCs

Tregs have been used for the treatment of autoimmune diseases because it modulates the autoimmune response by immune suppression. A number of mouse models demonstrated that Tregs are potent inhibitors of polyclonal T cell activation [52]. This Treg-mediated suppression is achieved by cytokine-independent and cell-contact-dependent mechanisms that require activation by TCR. When its cognate Ag activates Tregs, they can suppress the conventional T cells within the immediate vicinity regardless of the specificity. In this phenomenon, Treg does not need to recognize any specific Ag; they exert their suppressive efforts by recognizing the Ag on APC. Thus, any autoimmune affected organ or tissue can be targeted without the knowledge of the causative Ag by using Tregs. By utilizing this procedure, the maximal therapeutic effect will not be achieved, as it is not Ag-specific. Polyclonal Tregs also inhibit a wide range of other immune cells such as B cells, DCs, and monocytes [53–55]. It has also been observed that polyclonal Tregs failed to reverse ongoing autoimmunity because Tregs require Ag specificity to home/be retained at the appropriate site and exert active suppression. Within a polyclonal population of Tregs, Ag specificity against autoantigen exists in a small proportion of cells, which is not sufficient to exert sufficient amount of suppression. Therefore, it is crucial to generate a large number of Ag-specific Tregs for adoptive immunotherapy to reverse the ongoing autoimmunity.

Since it has been established that Tregs are the most potent to suppress the overactivity of hyperactive T cells, our approach was to generate a large number of Ag-specific Tregs from iPSCs. It is already published that hematopoietic stem cells (HSCs) and ESCs are able to differentiate into T cells in an *in vitro* culture system and we have utilized a similar approach to test whether iPSCs could follow the same trend [6, 56]. In that study, mouse iPSCs were cocultured with Notch ligand expressing bone marrow stromal cell line (OP9-DL1) as Notch ligand signaling is essential for T lineage differentiation [57]. At different days of cell culture, iPSCs were collected and evaluated for morphology, cell surface Ag, and their functional ability. It is found that iPSC-derived cells differentiated from stem-like cells to T cell-like cells, expressing T cell surface markers. Morphologically, dome-like stem cell colony was transformed to grape-like colony, which is a characteristic of lymphoid cells. iPSCs usually express CD117 and Nanog surface markers. After differentiation, the cells stopped expressing stem cell-like markers and expressed T cell markers such as CD4 and CD8. *In vitro* differentiated cells were also tested for their functional ability and it is found that they secrete IL-2 and IFN-α upon stimulation with anti-CD3 and anti-CD28 antibodies.

Since we could differentiate iPSCs into functional T cells, we proceeded to generate Ag-specific Tregs. First, we generated a construct called MiDR-TCR-FoxP3 where ovalbumin $(OVA)_{323-339}$ specific TCR OTII and FoxP3 were cloned into MiDR vector (**Figure 1**).

MiDR-TCR-FoxP3 vector was retrovirally transduced into mouse iPSCs and cocultured onto with OP9-DL1-DL4-I-A^b in the presence of recombinant cytokines of rIL-7 and rFLt3L. TCR and FoxP3 gene-transduced iPSCs were checked for differentiation by observing their morphological change. We found that iPSCs differentiated into mesoderm-like cells, and were associated with nonadherent grape-like clusters. On day 22 of culture, lymphocyte-like cell Spread fully across the plate (**Figure 2**).

In vitro cocultured cells were analyzed for cell surface markers. We found that the iPSC-derived cells substantially expressed CD3- and Ag-specific TCR, two T cell markers. The

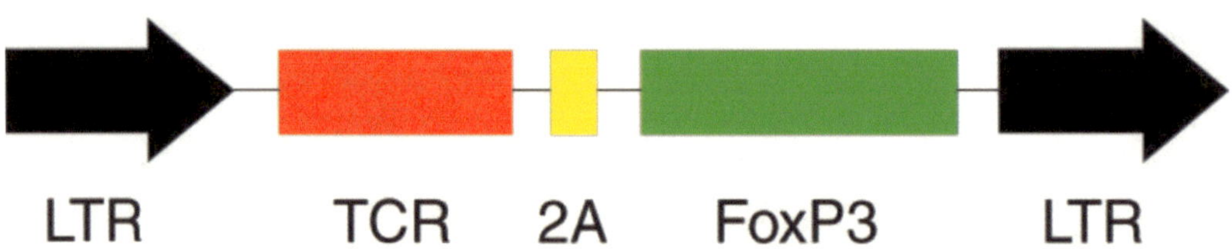

Figure 1. Generation of MiDR-TCR-FoxP3 retroviral construct. Schematic representation of the retrovirus construct MiDR-TCR-FoxP3 expressing OVA-specific TCR and FoxP3. Ψ, packaging signal; 2A, picornavirus self-cleaving 2A sequence; LTR, long terminal repeats.

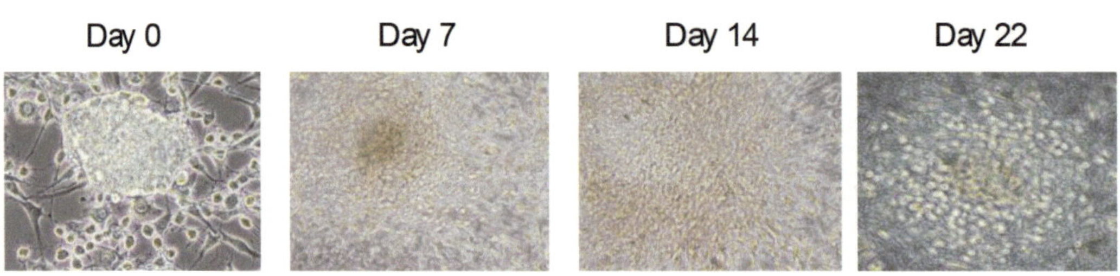

Figure 2. Morphology of Treg differentiation on days 0, 7, 14, and 22. The TCR/FoxP3 gene-transduced iPSCs were cocultured with OP9 stromal cell expressing Notch ligands DL1, DL4, and I-A^b in the presence of rIL-7 and r-Flt3L. Morphology was visualized under a microscope.

http://dx.doi.org/10.5772/66909

$CD3^+TCRV\beta5^+$ population expressed CD4. Most of the $CD3^+TCRV\beta5^+CD4^+$ cells expressed CD25, CD127, and CTLA-4, which are typically expressed at elevated levels in naturally occurring Tregs (iTregs) [58]. Subsequently, we also investigated the functional capability of iPSC-derived Ag-specific Tregs. After adoptive transfer, $CD4^+FoxP3^+$ Tregs were isolated from pancreatic lymph nodes and checked for expression of two suppressive cytokines, IL-10 and TGFβ. The result showed that significant amount of IL-10 and TGFβ were secreted by Tregs that supported that iPSC-derived Tregs are functional.

8. Utilization of iPSC-derived Tregs for the treatments of autoimmune diabetes

We developed a mouse model for autoimmune diabetes by crossing B6 mOVA transgenic (Tg) mice with OT I TCR Tg mice. In B6 mOVA Tg mice, membrane bound form of OVA expressed in the pancreatic islet β cells and the renal proximal tubular cells [59]. Once they are interbred, the resulting mice will be B6 mOVA-OT I where T cells from OT1 Tg mice will be directed to the pancreas as the pancreas expressed OVA autoantigen. The OT I OVA-specific T cells will begin to target and destroy pancreatic islet cells and mice will subsequently develop diabetes. Once pups reached 8 weeks, blood sugar level was measured and it was observed that only 30% mice developed diabetes. Subsequently, OT I Tg T cells were further triggered by injecting vaccinia virus expressing OVA (VV-OVA) into the mice. After vaccinia immunization, 100% mice developed diabetes with more urine discharge. After confirmation of disease developed in mice, we injected iPSC-derived Tregs into the mice. One-week post cell transfer, we checked the blood glucose level and found that more than 80% of the mice had reduced glucose level in their blood. Mice were sacrificed for histological evaluation. Pancreas were isolated from treated and untreated mice and it was observed that inflammation was markedly decreased in iPSC-derived Treg-transfer mice compare to untreated mice (**Figure 3**).

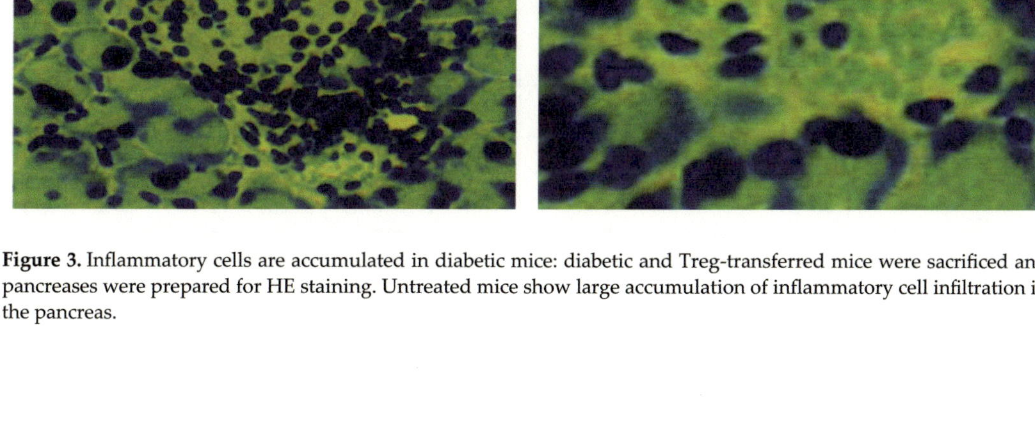

Figure 3. Inflammatory cells are accumulated in diabetic mice: diabetic and Treg-transferred mice were sacrificed and pancreases were prepared for HE staining. Untreated mice show large accumulation of inflammatory cell infiltration in the pancreas.

Further analysis was done to check the islet destruction in iPSC-derived Treg-transfer and nontransfer mice. Islet sizes were markedly reduced in nontransfer mice, whereas islet sizes were normal in iPSC-derived Treg-transfer mice (**Figure 4**).

We investigated the mechanisms of how iPSCs-derived Tregs controlled blood sugar levels and prevented the destruction of islet in autoimmune diabetes mice. Adhesion molecule

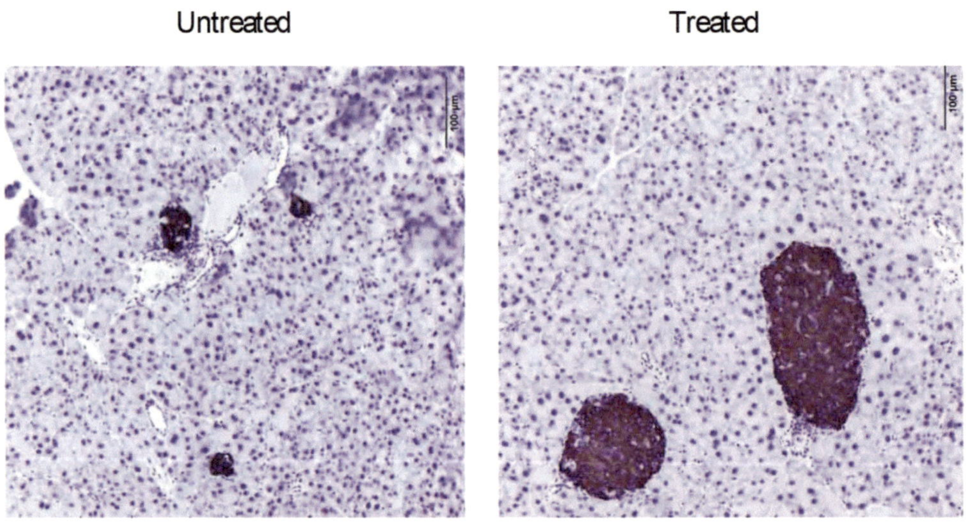

Figure 4. Islet size and numbers were reduced in diabetic mice. Diabetic and Treg-transferred mice were sacrificed and their Pancreas were stained with insulin to detect the beta cell. In diabetic mice, islets size and number were reduced markedly, whereas islet size and numbers were normal in Treg-transferred mice.

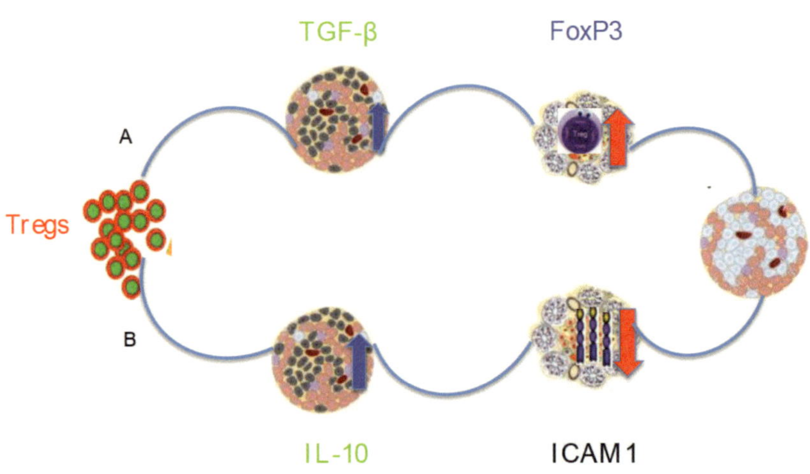

Figure 5. Stem cell-derived OVA-specific Tregs were adoptively transferred into diabetic mice. (A) Tregs induced the expression of TGF-β into the destructed islet leading to increase the expression of intra-islet FoxP3 that protected the islet from further destruction. (B) Tregs induced the expression of IL-10 into the destructed islet leading to reduce the expression of ICAM1 that prevented the migration of $CD8^+$ T cells into the destructed islet and protected the islet from further destruction.

http://dx.doi.org/10.5772/66909

ICAM1 is important for targeting autoreactive $CD8^+$ T cells into the pancreatic islet [32]. We determined the expression of ICAM1 into the pancreatic lymph nodes, and found that ICAM1 expression was dramatically increased in diabetic mice. Conversely, its expression was markedly reduced in iPSC-derived Treg-transfer mice. Previously, we have showed that iPSC-derived Tregs were able to secret IL-10 and TGF-β. Therefore, expression of TGF-β by iPSC-derived Tregs into the islet increased the intra-islet FoxP3 expression that protected the islet from further destruction. Moreover, IL-10 secreted by the Tregs reduced the expression of ICAM1, which prevented the migration of autoreactive $CD8^+$ T cell into the damaged islet and prevented further destruction of the islet (**Figure 5**).

9. Conclusion

PSCs have the ability to differentiate into Ag-specific Tregs and they are also found to be similar morphologically and functionally to iTregs. However, in autoimmune diabetes, it is important to mitigate the disease by increasing the activity of islet cells or preventing their destruction from autoreactive T cells. In our study, iPSC-derived Tregs were successful in reducing the blood sugar level and restoration of the islet size. By utilizing the knowledge from iPSC differentiation, We will be able to generate Ag-specific T cells that are more closely associated with the development of autoimmune diabetes. It is already known that heat shock proteins (HSPs) are an islet tissue-associated auto-Ag and involved in the islet cell destruction of T1D [60]. HSPs can modulate chronic inflammatory diseases and can be a target of immunotherapy of T1D. In our preliminary study, we checked the expression of HSPs in our diabetes model and found that diabetic mice substantially expressed HSPs. Therefore, it will be ideal to generate HSP-specific Tregs from PSCs for the treatment of autoimmune diabetes. For this study, HSP-specific TCR needs to be genetically processed and cloned into a viral vector to be retrovirally transduced into PSCs and follow the general protocol to allow for *in vitro* differentiation for the development of HSP-specific Tregs. In recent years, not only our efforts in utilizing PSC derived T cells for therapeutic purposes, but also other groups have made considerable efforts in understanding the PSC function in hematopoietic development. PSCs also could be differentiated into DCs, NK cells, and B cells. Consequently, by using patient-derived iPSCs, autoantigen-specific Tregs could be generated to specifically treat diabetic patients.

Acknowledgements

This project is funded, in part, under grants with the National Institute of Health Grant R01AI121180, R21AI109239, and K18CA151798, American Diabetes Association 1-16-IBS-281, and the Pennsylvania Department of Health using Tobacco Settlement Funds.

Author details

Mohammad Haque, Praneet Sandhu, Swetha Ravi, Sravya Kurapati and Jianxun Song*

*Address all correspondence to: jsong2@hmc.psu.edu

The Pennsylvania State University College of Medicine, Hershey, PA, USA

References

[1] Alexandropoulos K, Danzl NM. Thymic epithelial cells: antigen presenting cells that regulate T cell repertoire and tolerance development. Immunol Res. 2012 Dec;54(1-3):177–90. PubMed PMID: 22454100.

[2] Goodnow CC, Vinuesa CG, Randall KL, Mackay F, Brink R. Control systems and decision making for antibody production. Nat Immunol. 2010 Aug;11(8):681–8. PubMed PMID: 20644574.

[3] Rajewsky K. Clonal selection and learning in the antibody system. Nature. 1996 Jun 27;381(6585):751–8. PubMed PMID: 8657279.

[4] Haque M, Song J, Fino K, Sandhu P, Wang Y, Ni B, et al. Melanoma Immunotherapy in mice using genetically engineered pluripotent stem cells. Cell Transplant. 2016;25(5):811–27. PubMed PMID: 26777320.

[5] Miao D, Yu L, Eisenbarth GS. Role of autoantibodies in type 1 diabetes. Front Biosci. 2007;12:1889–98. PubMed PMID: 17127428.

[6] Haque M, Song J, Fino K, Sandhu P, Song X, Lei F, et al. Stem cell-derived tissue-associated regulatory T cells ameliorate the development of autoimmunity. Sci Rep. 2016;6:20588. PubMed PMID: 26846186. Pubmed Central PMCID: PMC4742827.

[7] Haque R, Lei F, Xiong X, Bian Y, Zhao B, Wu Y, et al. Programming of regulatory T cells from pluripotent stem cells and prevention of autoimmunity. J Immunol. 2012;189(3):1228–36. PubMed PMID: 22732595. Pubmed Central PMCID: 3401327.

[8] Fagot-Campagna A, Pettitt DJ, Engelgau MM, Burrows NR, Geiss LS, Valdez R, et al. Type 2 diabetes among North American children and adolescents: an epidemiologic review and a public health perspective. J Pediatr. 2000;136(5):664–72. PubMed PMID: 10802501.

[9] Anjos SM, Tessier MC, Polychronakos C. Association of the cytotoxic T lymphocyte-associated antigen 4 gene with type 1 diabetes: evidence for independent effects of two polymorphisms on the same haplotype block. J Clin Endocrinol Metab. 2004;89(12):6257–65. PubMed PMID: 15579786.

[10] Sanchez-Fueyo A, Sandner S, Habicht A, Mariat C, Kenny J, Degauque N, et al. Specificity of CD4+CD25+ regulatory T cell function in alloimmunity. J Immunol. 2006;176(1):329–34. PubMed PMID: 16365425. Pubmed Central PMCID: PMC2841032.

[11] Holt RI. Diagnosis, epidemiology and pathogenesis of diabetes mellitus: an update for psychiatrists. Br J Psychiatry Suppl. 2004;47:S55–63. PubMed PMID: 15056594.

[12] Hamalainen AM, Knip M. Autoimmunity and familial risk of type 1 diabetes. Curr Diab Rep. 2002;2(4):347–53. PubMed PMID: 12643195.

[13] Imagawa A, Hanafusa T, Tamura S, Moriwaki M, Itoh N, Yamamoto K, et al. Pancreatic biopsy as a procedure for detecting in situ autoimmune phenomena in type 1 diabetes:

close correlation between serological markers and histological evidence of cellular autoimmunity. Diabetes. 2001;50(6):1269–73. PubMed PMID: 11375326.

[14] Knip M, Ilonen J, Mustonen A, Akerblom HK. Evidence of an accelerated B-cell destruction in HLA-Dw3/Dw4 heterozygous children with type 1 (insulin-dependent) diabetes. Diabetologia. 1986;29(6):347–51. PubMed PMID: 3527834.

[15] Aly TA, Ide A, Jahromi MM, Barker JM, Fernando MS, Babu SR, et al. Extreme genetic risk for type 1A diabetes. Proc Natl Acad Sci U S A. 2006;103(38):14074–9. PubMed PMID: 16966600. Pubmed Central PMCID: PMC1563993.

[16] Dahms WT. An update in diabetes mellitus. Pediatr Dent. 1991;13(2):79–82. PubMed PMID: 1831890.

[17] Gill RG, Haskins K. Molecular mechanisms underlying diabetes and other autoimmune diseases. Immunol Today. 1993;14(2):49–51. PubMed PMID: 8095390.

[18] Boitard C, Yasunami R, Dardenne M, Bach JF. T cell-mediated inhibition of the transfer of autoimmune diabetes in NOD mice. J Exp Med. 1989;169(5):1669–80. PubMed PMID: 2523954. Pubmed Central PMCID: PMC2189316.

[19] Fowell D, McKnight AJ, Powrie F, Dyke R, Mason D. Subsets of CD4+ T cells and their roles in the induction and prevention of autoimmunity. Immunol Rev. 1991;123:37–64. PubMed PMID: 1684782.

[20] Tan T, Xiang Y, Chang C, Zhou Z. Alteration of regulatory T cells in type 1 diabetes mellitus: a comprehensive review. Clin Rev Allergy Immunol. 2014;47(2):234–43. PubMed PMID: 25086642.

[21] Mills KH. Regulatory T cells: friend or foe in immunity to infection? Nat Rev Immunol. 2004;4(11):841–55. PubMed PMID: 15516964.

[22] Sakaguchi S, Yamaguchi T, Nomura T, Ono M. Regulatory T cells and immune tolerance. Cell. 2008;133(5):775–87. PubMed PMID: 18510923.

[23] Wing K, Sakaguchi S. Regulatory T cells exert checks and balances on self-tolerance and autoimmunity. Nat Immunol. 2010;11(1):7–13. PubMed PMID: 20016504.

[24] Passerini L, Di Nunzio S, Gregori S, Gambineri E, Cecconi M, Seidel MG, et al. Functional type 1 regulatory T cells develop regardless of FOXP3 mutations in patients with IPEX syndrome. Eur J Immunol. 2011;41(4):1120–31. PubMed PMID: 21400500. Pubmed Central PMCID: PMC3107421.

[25] Salomon B, Lenschow DJ, Rhee L, Ashourian N, Singh B, Sharpe A, et al. B7/CD28 costimulation is essential for the homeostasis of the CD4+CD25+ immunoregulatory T cells that control autoimmune diabetes. Immunity. 2000;12(4):431–40. PubMed PMID: 10795741.

[26] Tang Q, Adams JY, Tooley AJ, Bi M, Fife BT, Serra P, et al. Visualizing regulatory T cell control of autoimmune responses in nonobese diabetic mice. Nat Immunol. 2006;7(1):83–92. PubMed PMID: 16311599. Pubmed Central PMCID: PMC3057888.

[27] Asnagli H, Martire D, Belmonte N, Quentin J, Bastian H, Boucard-Jourdin M, et al. Type 1 regulatory T cells specific for collagen type II as an efficient cell-based therapy in arthritis. Arthritis Res Ther. 2014;16(3):R115. PubMed PMID: 24886976. Pubmed Central PMCID: PMC4075412.

[28] Huygens C, Lienart S, Dedobbeleer O, Stockis J, Gauthy E, Coulie PG, et al. Lysosomal-associated transmembrane protein 4B (LAPTM4B) decreases transforming growth factor beta1 (TGF-beta1) production in human regulatory T cells. J Biol Chem. 2015;290(33):20105–16. PubMed PMID: 26126825. Pubmed Central PMCID: PMC4536422.

[29] Peng Y, Laouar Y, Li MO, Green EA, Flavell RA. TGF-beta regulates in vivo expansion of Foxp3-expressing CD4+CD25+ regulatory T cells responsible for protection against diabetes. Proc Natl Acad Sci U S A. 2004;101(13):4572–7. PubMed PMID: 15070759. Pubmed Central PMCID: PMC384788.

[30] Calderon B, Carrero JA, Miller MJ, Unanue ER. Entry of diabetogenic T cells into islets induces changes that lead to amplification of the cellular response. Proc Natl Acad Sci U S A. 2011;108(4):1567–72. PubMed PMID: 21220309. Pubmed Central PMCID: PMC3029718.

[31] Linn T, Strate C, Federlin K, Papaccio G. Intercellular adhesion molecule-1 (ICAM-1) expression in the islets of the non-obese diabetic and low-dose streptozocin-treated mouse. Histochemistry. 1994;102(4):317–21. PubMed PMID: 7843994.

[32] Battaglia M, Stabilini A, Draghici E, Migliavacca B, Gregori S, Bonifacio E, et al. Induction of tolerance in type 1 diabetes via both CD4+CD25+ T regulatory cells and T regulatory type 1 cells. Diabetes. 2006;55(6):1571–80. PubMed PMID: 16731819.

[33] Roncarolo MG, Battaglia M, Gregori S. The role of interleukin 10 in the control of autoimmunity. J Autoimmun. 2003;20(4):269–72. PubMed PMID: 12791310.

[34] Peterson RA. Regulatory T-cells: diverse phenotypes integral to immune homeostasis and suppression. Toxicol Pathol. 2012;40(2):186–204. PubMed PMID: 22222887.

[35] Venigalla RK, Guttikonda PJ, Eckstein V, Ho AD, Sertel S, Lorenz HM, et al. Identification of a human Th1-like IFNgamma-secreting Treg subtype deriving from effector T cells. J Autoimmun. 2012;39(4):377–87. PubMed PMID: 22824211.

[36] Walker LS. Treg and CTLA-4: two intertwining pathways to immune tolerance. J Autoimmun. 2013;45:49–57. PubMed PMID: 23849743. Pubmed Central PMCID: PMC3989116.

[37] Brusko TM, Putnam AL, Bluestone JA. Human regulatory T cells: role in autoimmune disease and therapeutic opportunities. Immunol Rev. 2008;223:371–90. PubMed PMID: 18613848.

[38] Sakaguchi S, Miyara M, Costantino CM, Hafler DA. FOXP3+ regulatory T cells in the human immune system. Nat Rev Immunol. 2010;10(7):490–500. PubMed PMID: 20559327.

[39] Battaglia M, Roncarolo MG. Immune intervention with T regulatory cells: past lessons and future perspectives for type 1 diabetes. Semin Immunol. 2011;23(3):182–94. PubMed PMID: 21831659.

[40] Putheti P, Pettersson A, Soderstrom M, Link H, Huang YM. Circulating CD4+CD25+ T regulatory cells are not altered in multiple sclerosis and unaffected by disease-modulating drugs. J Clin Immunol. 2004;24(2):155–61. PubMed PMID: 15024182.

[41] de Kleer IM, Wedderburn LR, Taams LS, Patel A, Varsani H, Klein M, et al. CD4+CD25bright regulatory T cells actively regulate inflammation in the joints of patients with the remitting form of juvenile idiopathic arthritis. Journal of immunology. 2004;172(10):6435–43. PubMed PMID: 15128835.

[42] von Herrath M, Sanda S, Herold K. Type 1 diabetes as a relapsing-remitting disease? Nat Rev Immunol. 2007;7(12):988–94. PubMed PMID: 17982429.

[43] Shapiro AM, Lakey JR, Ryan EA, Korbutt GS, Toth E, Warnock GL, et al. Islet transplantation in seven patients with type 1 diabetes mellitus using a glucocorticoid-free immunosuppressive regimen. N Engl J Med. 2000;343(4):230–8. PubMed PMID: 10911004.

[44] Zalzman M, Anker-Kitai L, Efrat S. Differentiation of human liver-derived, insulin-producing cells toward the beta-cell phenotype. Diabetes. 2005;54(9):2568–75. PubMed PMID: 16123344.

[45] Russ HA, Ravassard P, Kerr-Conte J, Pattou F, Efrat S. Epithelial-mesenchymal transition in cells expanded in vitro from lineage-traced adult human pancreatic beta cells. PLoS One. 2009;4(7):e6417. PubMed PMID: 19641613. Pubmed Central PMCID: PMC2712769.

[46] Maeda Y, Nishikawa H, Sugiyama D, Ha D, Hamaguchi M, Saito T, et al. Detection of self-reactive CD8(+) T cells with an anergic phenotype in healthy individuals. Science. 2014;346(6216):1536–40. PubMed PMID: 25525252.

[47] Okita K, Ichisaka T, Yamanaka S. Generation of germline-competent induced pluripotent stem cells. Nature. 2007;448(7151):313–7. PubMed PMID: 17554338.

[48] Huangfu D, Osafune K, Maehr R, Guo W, Eijkelenboom A, Chen S, et al. Induction of pluripotent stem cells from primary human fibroblasts with only Oct4 and Sox2. Nat Biotechnol. 2008;26(11):1269–75. PubMed PMID: 18849973.

[49] Okita K, Nakagawa M, Hyenjong H, Ichisaka T, Yamanaka S. Generation of mouse induced pluripotent stem cells without viral vectors. Science. 2008;322(5903):949–53. PubMed PMID: 18845712.

[50] Giorgetti A, Montserrat N, Rodriguez-Piza I, Azqueta C, Veiga A, Izpisua Belmonte JC. Generation of induced pluripotent stem cells from human cord blood cells with only two factors: Oct4 and Sox2. Nat Protoc. 2010;5(4):811–20. PubMed PMID: 20360773.

[51] Maehr R, Chen S, Snitow M, Ludwig T, Yagasaki L, Goland R, et al. Generation of pluripotent stem cells from patients with type 1 diabetes. Proc Natl Acad Sci U S A. 2009;106(37):15768–73. PubMed PMID: 19720998. Pubmed Central PMCID: PMC2735559.

[52] Thornton AM, Shevach EM. CD4+CD25+ immunoregulatory T cells suppress polyclonal T cell activation in vitro by inhibiting interleukin 2 production. J Exp Med. 1998;188(2):287–96. PubMed PMID: 9670041. Pubmed Central PMCID: PMC2212461.

[53] Fallarino F, Grohmann U, Hwang KW, Orabona C, Vacca C, Bianchi R, et al. Modulation of tryptophan catabolism by regulatory T cells. Nat Immunol. 2003;4(12):1206–12. PubMed PMID: 14578884.

[54] Lim HW, Hillsamer P, Banham AH, Kim CH. Cutting edge: direct suppression of B cells by CD4+ CD25+ regulatory T cells. J Immunol. 2005;175(7):4180–3. PubMed PMID: 16177055.

[55] Tiemessen MM, Jagger AL, Evans HG, van Herwijnen MJ, John S, Taams LS. CD4+CD25+Foxp3+ regulatory T cells induce alternative activation of human monocytes/macrophages. Proc Natl Acad Sci U S A. 2007;104(49):19446–51. PubMed PMID: 18042719. Pubmed Central PMCID: PMC2148309.

[56] Lei F, Haque R, Weiler L, Vrana KE, Song J. T lineage differentiation from induced pluripotent stem cells. Cell Immunol. 2009;260(1):1–5. PubMed PMID: 19811778.

[57] Dai B, Wang P. In vitro differentiation of adult bone marrow progenitors into antigen-specific CD4 helper T cells using engineered stromal cells expressing a notch ligand and a major histocompatibility complex class II protein. Stem Cells Dev. 2009;18(2):235–45. PubMed PMID: 18680390. Pubmed Central PMCID: PMC2656584.

[58] Rubtsov YP, Niec RE, Josefowicz S, Li L, Darce J, Mathis D, et al. Stability of the regulatory T cell lineage in vivo. Science. 2010;329(5999):1667–71. PubMed PMID: 20929851. Pubmed Central PMCID: PMC4262151.

[59] Kurts C, Heath WR, Carbone FR, Allison J, Miller JF, Kosaka H. Constitutive class I-restricted exogenous presentation of self antigens in vivo. J Exp Med. 1996;184(3):923–30. PubMed PMID: 9064352. Pubmed Central PMCID: PMC2192761.

[60] Sarikonda G, Sachithanantham S, Miller JF, Pagni PP, Coppieters KT, von Herrath M. The Hsp60 peptide p277 enhances anti-CD3 mediated diabetes remission in non-obese diabetic mice. J Autoimmun. 2015;59:61–6. PubMed PMID: 25772283.

Chapter 3

Early- Versus Late-Onset Type 1 Diabetes: Two Different Pathophysiological Subtypes with Implications for Therapy

Willem M. Kühtreiber, Miriam Davis and
Denise L. Faustman

Additional information is available at the end of the chapter

http://dx.doi.org/10.5772/65598

Abstract

Insulin, as measured by C-peptide, is produced for decades after onset of type 1 diabetes, and even very low levels of C-peptide have clinical significance. In this chapter we show that two distinct pathophysiological subtypes of type 1 diabetic subjects can be distinguished. Early-onset diabetic subjects (≤20 years) have rapid loss of C-peptide, whereas late-onset diabetic subjects (>20 years) have slower C-peptide declines over decades. Early-onset diabetics have significantly lower levels of persistent autoreactive CD8+ T cells than do late-onset diabetic subjects. In late-onset disease, robust production of autoreactive T-cells occurs even in the absence of C-peptide. Metabolomics analysis reveals frequent differences between the two subtypes of subjects in the levels of amino acids, carbohydrates, cofactors, lipids, peptides, and xenobiotics. There are statistically significant differences related to protective islet functions, islet health, development, blood sugar control, and regulation of exocrine pancreas function. Taken together these findings suggest that pancreas pathobiology, as well as durability of abnormal T-cell response should be considered in immune targeting treatments. Therapies aimed at immune defects alone are likely to work best in late-onset diabetics. Therapies aimed at islet cell preservation in early-onset diabetic subjects likely have greater efficacy if administered shortly after disease onset.

Keywords: type 1 diabetes, C-peptide, metabolomics, autoreactive T-cells, therapy, type 1 diabetic subtypes, early-onset diabetes, late-onset diabetes, metabolites

1. Introduction

This chapter summarizes the evidence supporting two distinct pathophysiological subtypes of type 1 diabetes (T1D) based on age of onset (AOO). The characterization of these two subtypes—early- versus late-onset—traces back to the finding that β-islet cells of the pancreas are still functional decades after disease onset. When first published in 2012 [1], this finding ran against conventional wisdom that all beta cells die within 2 years of onset and that type 1 diabetics usually have an absolute deficiency of insulin [2]. Instead, low levels of C-peptide, which is co-secreted with insulin and thus serves as the best measure of endogenous insulin secretion, persist for decades after disease onset. Confirmation of the study by Wang and colleagues came from several studies [3–8], showing that 80% of people with long-standing diabetes have low but detectable levels of C-peptide upon stimulation with oral glucose [9]. These studies were made possible by new ultrasensitive C-peptide assays with detection limits of 1.5–5.0 pmol/L. Older C-peptide assay typically only detected to 40–50 pmol/L. The low levels of C-peptide were indicative of intact β-islet cell function according to assays showing that C-peptide levels rose in response to hyperglycemia or a mixed-meal stimulus [1, 4, 5]. Intact β-islet cell function in long-standing disease suggests that β-islet cells are either regenerating or evading immune attack.

What's more is that these low levels of C-peptide or any persistent C-peptide have clinical significance. They are associated with fewer diabetic complications (e.g., nephropathy, neuropathy, foot ulcers, and retinopathy), better metabolic control via HbA1c, and prevention of hypoglycemia [7, 10–12]. The finding of C-peptide persistence and its clinical significance paved the way for an examination of the pathophysiological differences between early- and late-onset type 1 diabetes.

2. Rate of C-peptide decline differs between early- and late-onset diabetes

Early-onset diabetics have a rapid loss of residual C-peptide, whereas late-onset diabetics have a slower rate of C-peptide decline, which occurs over decades [1, 6, 8]. Here, we confirm this finding with one of the largest patient samples to date of fasting C-peptides.

Cross-sectional data from 1958 long-term type 1 diabetics, who were recruited to the Massachusetts General Hospital, show the gradual decades-long decline in fasting C-peptide secretion from the pancreatic islets (**Figure 1A**). The rate of decline in this group varied according to age of onset, with early-onset diabetics (n = 1063) showing a rapid decline and late-onset (n = 895) showing a slow decline (**Figure 1B**, left and right panels). The difference in C-peptide secretion between early-onset and late-onset subjects is statistically significant ($p <$ 0.001). Detecting low fasting C-peptide levels during the decades-long decay is possible

http://dx.doi.org/10.5772/65598

because of the improved detection limit with ultrasensitive ELISA[1] of only 1.5 pmol/L, which is significantly lower than older C-peptide assays with detection limits in the 40–50 pmol/L range [1]. The remainder of the chapter delves into the pathophysiological basis of this finding, using an assay for autoreactive CD8+ T lymphocytes (hereinafter referred to as autoreactive T-cells) and using metabolomics, the study of small molecules from intermediate metabolism.

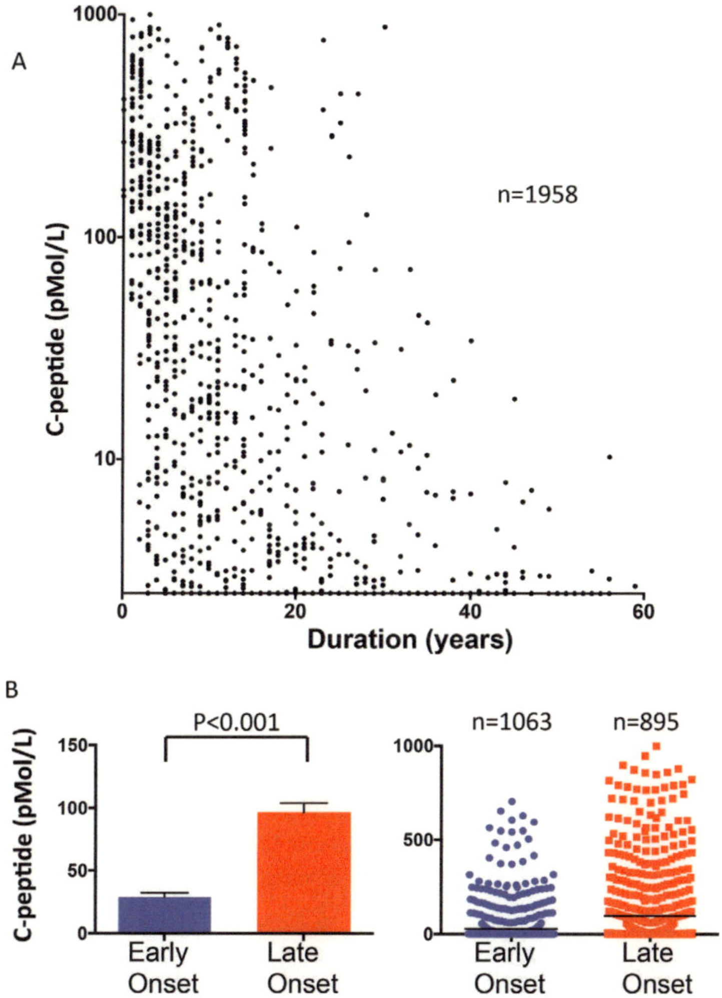

Figure 1. The decades-long persistence of C-peptide in patients with type 1 diabetes (n = 1958) and the more rapid fall in C-peptide levels with younger age of onset. (A) There is a gradual, decade-long decline in C-peptide detectable with an ultrasensitive assay. (B) The decline in C-peptide levels is related to the age of onset of the disease. Data are stratified by early- (left, blue) or late-onset diabetes (right, red). p Values were calculated using a Mann-Whitney U test (Wilcoxon rank-sum test), and the data are represented as mean ± SEM $p < 0.001$. The left panel depicts the large difference in mean C-peptide, whereas the right panel shows the same data according to individual data points.

[1] Cat. No 10-1141-01, Mercodia AB (Uppsala, Sweden). The assay was calibrated against the International Reference Reagent for C-peptide (IRR C-peptide 84/510; a WHO standard) and listed with the US Food and Drug Administration as Class I IVD device.

3. Levels of autoreactive T-cells differ between early- and late-onset diabetes

Here, we provide evidence that early-onset diabetics (≤20 years of age) have a significantly lower level of autoreactive T-cells than do late-onset diabetics (>20 years of age). We studied autoreactive T-cells in a subset (n = 178) of our sample (n = 1958) using a peptide-major histocompatibility complex class I (pMHC-I) multimer technique (fluorochrome-conjugated and peptide-loaded major histocompatibility complex class I multimers) in conjunction with flow cytometry. Two diabetes-specific peptides for autoreactive T-cell detection were used, i.e., peptide sequences from epitopes of pancreatic beta cells, islet-specific glucose-6-phosphatase catalytic subunit-related protein (IGRP) or insulin B chain (InsB) (tetramers were purchased from Beckman Coulter, Fullerton, CA, whereas dextramers were a generous gift from Immudex, Copenhagen, Denmark). For the IGRP peptide, pMHC-I was loaded with the peptide sequence for amino acids 228–236 (LNIDLLWSV). For the InsB peptide, pMHC-I was loaded with the peptide sequence corresponding to amino acids 10–18 (HLVEALYLV). For background fluorescence of T-cells, a matched negative (neg) HLA class I structure was loaded with an irrelevant peptide. The peptide sequence of the negative controls is kept proprietary by the companies but does not occur on mammalian cells (Beckman Coulter, Immudex). Using these methods, type 1 diabetics for decades after diagnosis have detectable levels of autoreactive T-cells measured with peptide-major histocompatibility complex class I (pMHC-I) multimers (**Figure 2**).

Type 1 diabetics were cross-sectionally studied for the presence or absence of autoreactive T-cells for decades after disease onset. The patients all had established type 1 diabetes (**Table 1**). Subjects had mean age of onset of 27.9 ± 1.6 years and a mean duration of diabetes of 14.9 ± 1.4 years. Typically, autoreactive T-cell detection studies are performed shortly after disease onset. However, because we wanted to know the association between prolonged C-peptide secretion and autoreactive T-cells, this study spanned decades of diabetes duration with simultaneous monitoring of C-peptide. Autoreactive T-cells were defined as samples staining with either IGRP or InsB MHC class I multimers. The data show that some long-standing diabetics have persistence of autoreactive T-cells decades after disease onset.

The type 1 diabetic subjects studied for autoreactive T-cells with pMHC-I multimers were divided into two groups, based on their status of early onset (n = 131, shown in blue) or late onset (n = 47), shown in red (**Figures 3** and **4**, **Table 1**). For each group, we determined the disease duration versus the serum C-peptide levels (**Figure 3A**). For each group, we also determined the presence of autoreactive T-cells versus disease duration (**Figure 4**). We once again observed that the decay of C-peptide secretion is faster in the early-onset group as compared to the late-onset group. For most subjects with early-onset, the C-peptide became undetectable within 10 years, whereas in the late-onset subjects, C-peptide lingered for decades (**Figure 3A**). The difference in C-peptide between the early-onset and late-onset was highly significant (C-peptide for early-onset 33.9 ± 5.4 pmol/L versus C-peptide for late-onset 98.6 ± 13.5 pmol/L (mean ± SEM; one-tailed Mann-Whitney U test $p < 0.0001$)).

http://dx.doi.org/10.5772/65598

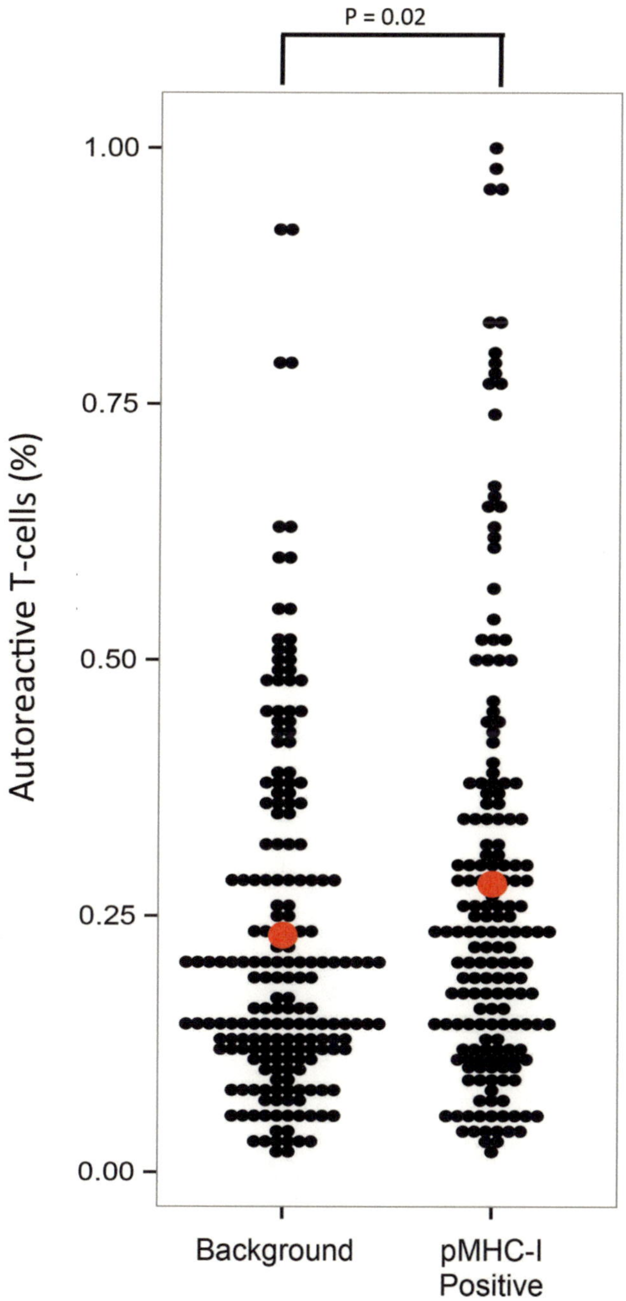

Figure 2. Type 1 diabetics for decades after diagnosis have detectable levels of autoreactive T-cells measured with peptide-major histocompatibility complex I (pMHC-I) multimers. Both insulin B and IGRP pMHC-I multimers were able to detect autoreactive CD8 T-cells of long-term diabetics. $n = 192$ samples for negative controls and $n = 178$ for samples stained for autoreactive cells. The means are represented by the large red dots. The background of 0.24% positive background fluorescence was used as the lower limits of detectability for the presence of pMHC-I multimers. Mann-Whitney U test shows a significant difference at $p = 0.02$.

	All	Early	Late
n	178	47	131
AOO (years)	27.9 ± 1.6	10.7 ± 1.2	34.7 ± 1.1
Duration (years)	14.9 ± 1.4	22.0 ± 2.6	11.3 ± 1.3
% Female	42.0%	46.2%	40.5%
C-peptide (pmol/L)	47.6 ± 14.3	3.8 ± 1.3	78.8 ± 18.9
Gad65 Ab (U/mL)	93.0 ± 12.0	84.7 ± 26.5	95.5 ± 13.5

All values are mean ± SEM.

Table 1. Clinical characteristics for early- and late-onset T1D.

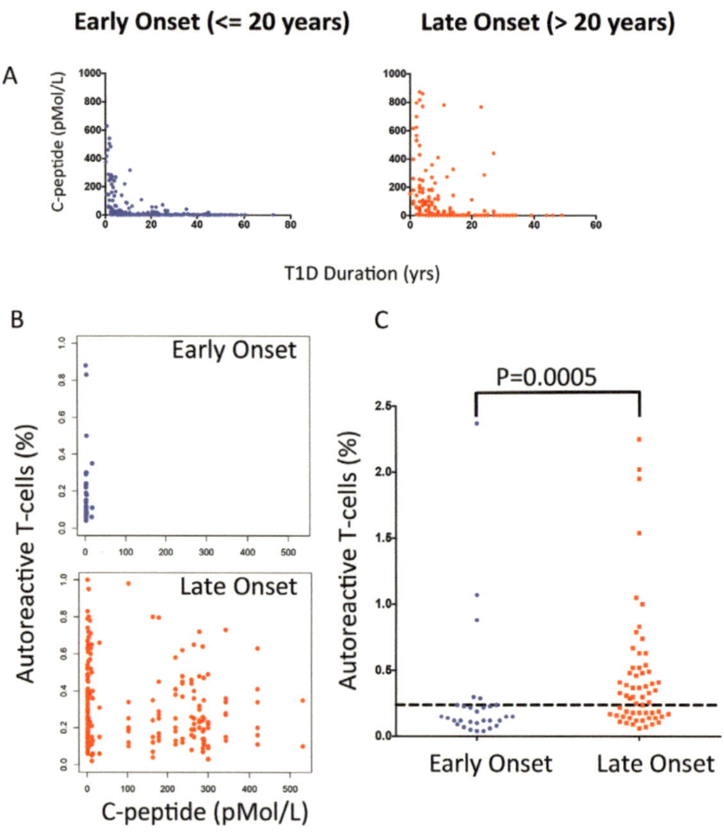

Figure 3. Early- and late-onset type 1 diabetics not only vary in the persistence of C-peptide but also dramatically vary by the presence or absence of autoreactive T-cells. (A) For this data set of early-onset diabetics ($n = 47$) and late-onset diabetics ($n = 131$), C-peptide decay continues to show prolonged presence exclusively in late-onset diabetes. (B) Late-onset diabetics have persistence of C-peptide and also the presence of abundant autoreactive T-cells. Early-onset diabetics have neither the persistence of C-peptide nor the presence of autoreactive cells. (C) At undetectable C-peptide levels in an ultrasensitive assay almost no autoreactive T-cells are detectable in early-onset subjects, but abundant autoreactive T-cells are present in late-onset diabetics. Mann-Whitney *U* test, $p = 0.0005$.

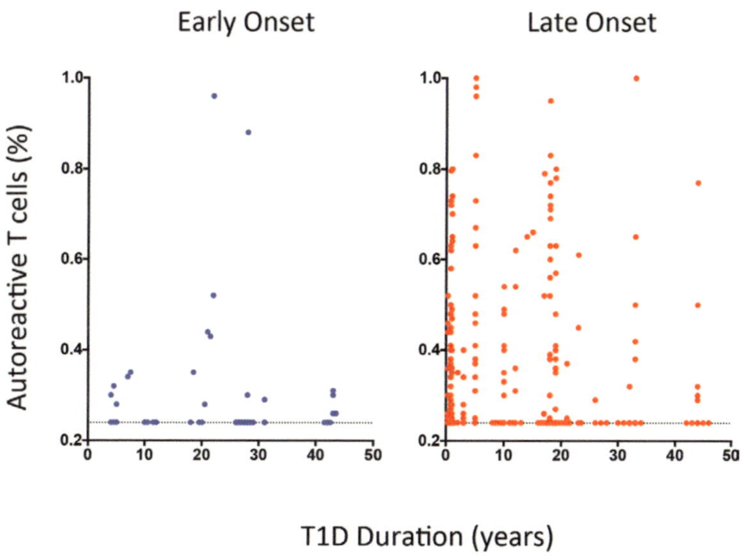

Figure 4. Relationship of diabetes disease duration and presence of autoreactive T-cells; comparison of early- and late-onset diabetes.

We then determined the levels of autoreactive T-cells in the early- and late-onset diabetic subjects using the pMHC-I multimer technique (**Figure 3B** and **C**). The early-onset group had little or no detectable C-peptide and little to no autoreactive T-cells. In contrast, the late-onset group frequently had large amounts of C-peptide coupled with large numbers of autoreactive T-cells. At first glance this seemed to make sense since the presence of islet activity in the pancreas is expected to be associated with the persistence of active CD8 autoimmunity. Also when we studied early- and late-onset subject pMHC-I autoreactive T-cells compared to disease duration, the early-onset diabetics had no relationship with duration and the presence or absence of T-cells. In contrast, late-onset diabetics had a decades-long decay in the presence of autoreactive T-cells (**Figure 4**).

But when early- and late-onset diabetics were compared when neither group had any detectable C-peptide, the late-onset diabetic subjects still continued to exhibit the abundant presence of autoreactive T-cells (**Figure 3B** and **C**, $p = 0.0005$). In marked contrast, when the early-onset diabetics were without detectable C-peptide, even when using an ultrasensitive C-peptide assay, almost no autoreactive T-cells were found in the early-onset cohorts. What are the possible explanations?

Our favored explanation is that autoreactive T-cells play a much more dominant role in disease etiology in late-onset than in early-onset disease. The massive abundance of detectable autoreactive T-cells in late-onset diabetics even without detectable C-peptide may reflect greater regenerative abilities of the pancreas, causing autoreactive T-cells to remain in the circulation. A trivial second explanation is that the two types of autoreactive T-cells measured, i.e., InsB and IGRP autoreactive T-cells, represent the dominant autoreactive epitopes in late-onset disease, but not in early-onset disease. Although C-peptide can now be detected to 1.5

pmol/L, this assay might still not be sensitive enough, and the T-cell assay is more sensitive for residual pancreatic activity, and that would also be an explanation for long-term autoreactive T-cells in late-onset diabetic subjects.

Why such non-detectable levels of autoreactive T-cells in early-onset diabetics? Primary pancreas defects unrelated to autoreactive T-cells may contribute to more rapid pancreatic islet failure in early-onset diabetics. The role of autoreactive T-cells may be less dominant in early-onset cases. Or as above, these early-onset diabetic subjects truly have no C-peptide and levels far below the sensitive assay levels of new C-peptide assays of 1.5 pmol/L.

4. Metabolomics differ between early- and late-onset diabetes

We studied metabolites in the serum of early-onset versus late-onset diabetics that might shed light on disease pathophysiology. Metabolomics was performed on two independently collected subject serum sets, referred to as serum set 1 and serum set 2, in order to verify findings. The subjects were two matched sets with 25 early- and 25 late-onset diabetic subjects with HbA1Cs in the same range. A total of 100 frozen serum samples were analyzed. The samples were sent for metabolic profiling to Metabolon (Durham, NC). Samples were extracted and prepared for analysis on Metabolon's integrated discovery platform that was based on a combination of gas and liquid chromatography techniques coupled with mass spectrometry for detection and identification. Metabolon's platform has met with considerable success in, among many studies, the identification of biomarkers of insulin resistance in subjects that are at risk of developing type 2 diabetes [13].

The clinical and biochemical characteristics of each serum set are shown in **Table 2**. The patient selections for each sample set were limited to subjects with disease duration of less than 25 years and a current age of less than 50 years to exclude kidney disease and other confounding factors in metabolism. We then statistically compared the data from early- versus late-onset diabetics and report only on those metabolites that were significantly different across both screens.

	AOO (years)	Age (years)	Duration (years)	C-peptide (pmol/mL)	HbA1C (%)	Female (%)
Serum set 1						
Early-onset	9.8 ± 0.7	23.3 ± 1.5	9.5 ± 1.2	40.5 ± 18.5	8.2 ± 0.4	32.0
Late-onset	35.8 ± 2.0	48.6 ± 2.3	8.4 ± 1.0	117.5 ± 43.5	7.2 ± 0.2	44.0
Serum set 2						
Early-onset	10.2 ± 0.7	16.8 ± 0.9	5.7 ± 0.9	87.9 ± 29.8	7.5 ± 0.2	36.0
Late-onset	32.8 ± 2.5	41.5 ± 2.3	7.7 ± 1.1	152.5 ± 50.6	6.7 ± 0.2	44.0

All values are mean ± SEM.

Table 2. Clinical characteristics of early- and late-onset diabetics for metabolomic assays .

Table 3 lists 30 metabolites that display statistically significant differences between early-onset and late-onset type 1 diabetes from both serum set 1 and serum set 2. These metabolites are found in diverse super pathway families, including amino acids, carbohydrates, cofactors and vitamins, lipids, peptides, and xenobiotics. **Table 3** also lists the subpathways. **Figure 5** graphs the same data according to the fold differences and also the direction, i.e., early- < late-onset or early- > late-onset. The data show that the fold differences were extremely similar for serum set 1 subjects and serum set 2 subjects and always in the same direction. The data trends were remarkably reproducible given that these were independently collected human samples.

Metabolite	Super pathway	Subpathway	*p* Serum set 1	*p* Serum set 2
Creatinine	Amino acid	Creatine metabolism	0.0206	0.034
N-acetyl-3-methylhistidine	Amino acid	Histidine metabolism	0.0018	0.0441
3-methylglutaconate	Amino acid	Leucine, isoleucine, and valine metabolism	0.0049	0.0216
N2-acetyllysine	Amino acid	Lysine metabolism	0.0429	0.0334
N-acetylphenylalanine	Amino acid	Phenylalanine and tyrosine metabolism	0.0092	0.0345
Spermidine	Amino acid	Polyamine metabolism	0.0458	0.0224
N-acetyltryptophan	Amino acid	Tryptophan metabolism	0.001	0.036
Pro-hydroxy-pro	Amino acid	Urea cycle: arginine and proline metabolism	1.06E−05	2.81E−09
Trans-4-hydroxyproline	Amino acid	Urea cycle: arginine and proline metabolism	0.001	3.00E−04
Glucuronate	Carbohydrate	Amino sugar metabolism	0.025	3.34E−08
Sucrose	Carbohydrate	Disaccharides and oligosaccharides	0.007	4.00E−04
Fructose	Carbohydrate	Fructose, mannose, and galactose metabolism	0.020	0.003
Sorbitol	Carbohydrate	Fructose, mannose, and galactose metabolism	0.001	0.001
Glucose	Carbohydrate	Glycolysis, gluconeogenesis, and pyruvate metabolism	0.003	0.044
Ascorbate (vitamin C)	Cofactors and vitamins	Ascorbate and aldarate metabolism	0.018	0.012
Trigonelline (N′-methylnicotinate)	Cofactors and vitamins	Nicotinate and nicotinamide metabolism	0.005	1.40E−06
Alpha-tocopherol (vitamin E)	Cofactors and vitamins	Tocopherol metabolism	0.001	0.002
Pyridoxate (vitamin B6)	Cofactors and	Vitamin B6 metabolism	0.002	0.014

Metabolite	Super pathway	Subpathway	*p* Serum set 1	*p* Serum set 2
	vitamins			
CMPF	Lipid	Fatty acid, dicarboxylate	0.000	0.001
Eicosapentaenoate (EPA)	Lipid	Polyunsaturated fatty acid (n3 and n6)	2.00E−04	0.002
Hyocholate	Lipid	Secondary bile acid metabolism	0.001	0.023
Taurodeoxycholate	Lipid	Secondary bile acid metabolism	0.011	0.047
Etiocholanolone glucuronide	Lipid	Steroid	0.021	0.002
Cholesterol	Lipid	Sterol	0.014	0.009
Leucylglycine	Peptide	Dipeptide	0.003	0.012
Valylglycine	Peptide	Dipeptide	0.001	2.75E−07
1,3-dimethylurate	Xenobiotics	Xanthine metabolism	0.010	0.004
1,3,7-trimethylurate	Xenobiotics	Xanthine metabolism	0.020	0.001
1,7-dimethylurate	Xenobiotics	Xanthine metabolism	0.024	0.009
Paraxanthine	Xenobiotics	Xanthine metabolism	0.032	0.007

Table 3. Early- versus late-onset T1D: metabolites with significant differences.

A subset of 7 out of 30 metabolites is important and is involved in pancreatic function (**Table 4**). In all cases, the pancreas-related metabolites were statistically different between early-onset and late-onset diabetic subjects.

Subjects with early- versus late-onset diabetes have varying levels of acetyllysine. Developing and proliferating insulin-secreting β-islet cells have augmented acetyltransferase activity related to growth and insulin secretion often through beta-cell–specific transcription factors BETA2 and PDX-1. High lysine deacetylase activity would be expected to increase the removal of acetyl groups from proteins. In our data the early-onset diabetics had lower levels of acetyllysine. Lysine deacetylase inhibitors protect β-islet cells by increasing the acetylation of proteins. In support of our observations, treatment data from the nonobese diabetic (NOD) mouse, an animal model of type 1 diabetes, shows that lysine deacetylase inhibition protects β-islet cells by increased acetylation of proteins [14]. Indeed, if lysine deacetylase inhibitors are brought forward to humans, their impact might be greater in early-onset diabetic subjects by conferring a presumed β-islet cell protective factor and restoring acetyllysine levels to higher levels.

Eicosapentaenoate (EPA), a metabolite of the polyunsaturated fatty acid metabolic pathway, was lower in early-onset type 1 diabetes and high in late-onset diabetics even exceeding the levels of control populations. Several studies support the concept that EPA improves insulin secretion in pancreatic islets [15, 16]. Since we found that EPA is lower in early-onset diabetes compared to late-onset diabetics, this again supports a more rapid disease progression in such individuals. It also suggests late-onset diabetic subjects could make EPA as a protective factor.

http://dx.doi.org/10.5772/65598

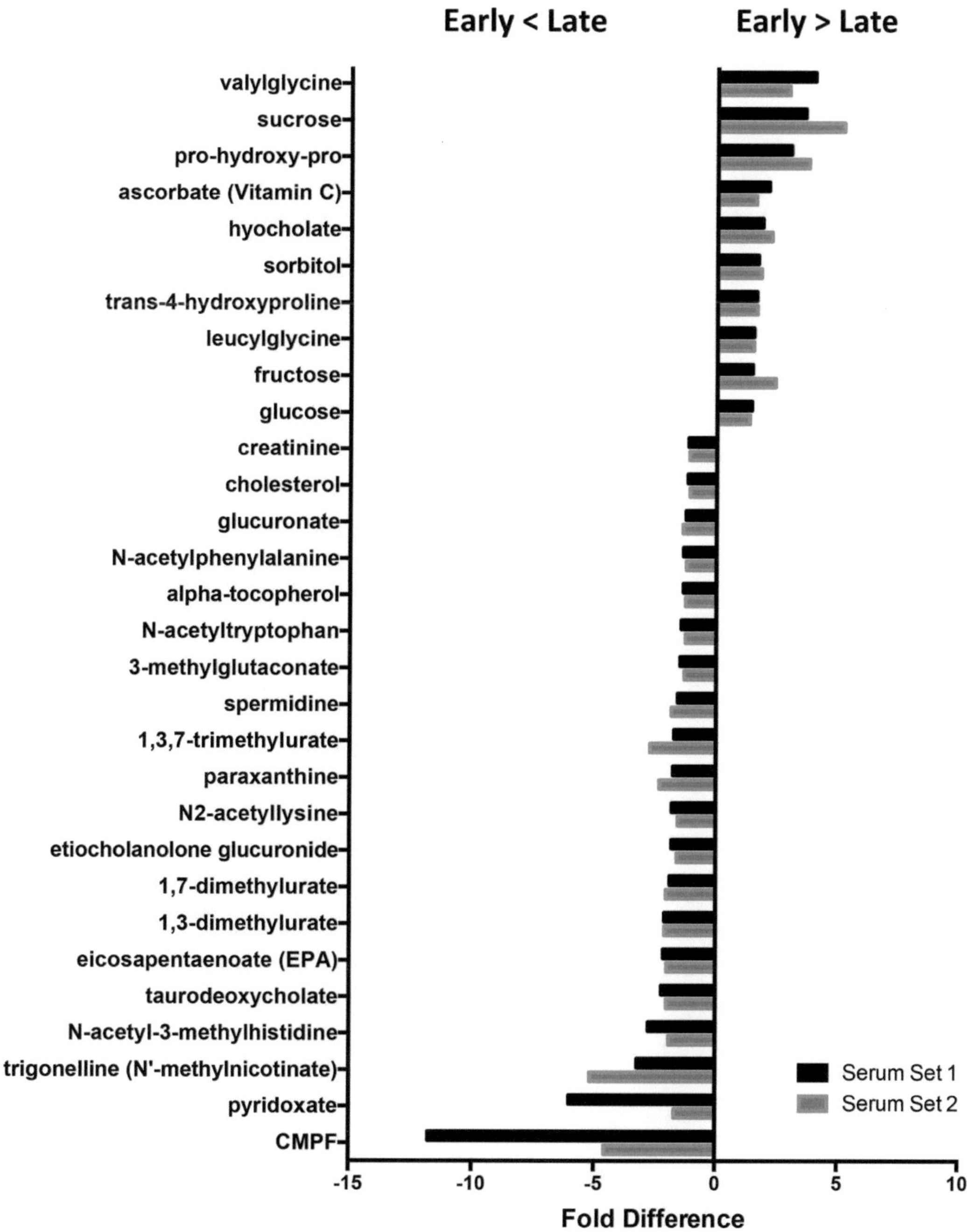

Figure 5. The over- and under-expression of metabolites associated with early- and late-onset diabetes. Shown is the ratio of metabolites in early- versus late-onset. For clarity, ratios between 0 and 1 were inverted (1/ratio) and made negative. Data are presented as rank order based on the magnitude of the statistically significant metabolic trends. Both sample sets demonstrate the tight reproducibility in the direction of the trends and also in the reproducibility of the magnitude of the derangements between early- and late-onset type 1 diabetics.

Metabolite	Pathway	Ratio early/ late (average of both screens)	Association with diabetes	References
N2-acetyllysine	Lysine metabolism	0.596	Diabetes induces lysine acetylation of intermediary metabolism enzymes in the kidney	Kosanam et al. [14]
Spermidine	Polyamine metabolism	0.588	Spermidine may decrease ER stress in pancreatic beta cells and may reduce apoptosis via activating AMPK-dependent autophagy pathway. Spermidine content is decreased in islets of old obese ob/ob mice. Polyamines such as spermidine increase the stability of insulin mRNA and are necessary for the maintenance of normal insulin and protein biosynthesis in islets	Tirupathi Pichiah et al [36]; Sjoholm et al. [23]; Welsh [21]; Welsh [22]
N-acetyltryptophan	Tryptophan metabolism	0.742	Suppresses rise in blood sugar and preserves insulin secretion in type 2; related to activity of intestinal bacteria	Wikoff et al. [17]
Glucuronate	Amino sugar metabolism	0.761	Elevated in diabetes. Glucuronate pathway is overactive in diabetes	Winegrad and Burden [25]
CMPF	Fatty acid, dicarboxylate metabolism	0.152	Elevated in diabetes. Causes beta-cell dysfunction	Nolan [26]; Prentice et al. [27]
Eicosapentaenoate (EPA)	Polyunsaturated fatty acid metabolism	0.480	Improves insulin secretion in pancreatic islets	Kato et al. [15]; Shimano et al. [16]
Taurodeoxycholate	Secondary bile acid metabolism	0.470	Involved in regulation of exocrine pancreas function	Riepl et al. [18]

Table 4. Early- versus late-onset diabetics: islet-, insulin-, and pancreas-related metabolites with significant differences.

N-acetyltryptophan was also observed to be lower in early-onset diabetics. N-acetyltryptophan suppresses rises in blood sugars and preserves insulin secretion in type 1 diabetes [17]. Abundant n-acetyltryptophan also can be produced by select gut bacteria and modulates

http://dx.doi.org/10.5772/65598

expression of proinflammatory genes and increases expression of anti-inflammatory genes possibly affecting the etiology of both early- and late-onset diabetes [17].

Taurodeoxycholate, a metabolite related to secondary bile acid metabolism, was more depressed in early-onset than late-onset diabetes. Previous evidence shows this metabolite is involved in the regulation of exocrine pancreas function [18]. Exocrine pancreatic dysfunction in type 1 diabetes is linked to a decrease in pancreatic volume, an observation of past reports [19]. Therefore, our findings again point to varying contributions of pancreas defects to T1D in early-onset subjects compared to late-onset diabetics.

Spermidine, a member of the polyamine metabolism, was decreased in early-onset diabetics and elevated in late-onset subjects. Past reports suggest type 1 diabetic subjects have reduced spermidine levels, and now our data suggests this deficiency is even more pronounced in early-onset diabetes [20]. Spermidine may decrease endoplasmic reticulum (ER) stress in pancreatic islet beta cells, is decreased in islets of obese-hyperglycemic ob/ob mice, and is also reported to reduce apoptosis via AMP-activated protein kinase (AMPK)-dependent autophagy pathways [21–24]. A deficiency in spermidine might accelerate disease onset.

Glucuronate, which was also lower in early-onset diabetes, is involved in amino sugar metabolism. Some reports characterize this metabolite as related to diabetic hyperglycemia [25]. Again this points to altered and varying levels between early- and late-onset subjects.

Lastly, the metabolite 3-carboxy-4-methyl-5-propyl-2-furanpropanoic acid (CMPF) was high in late-onset diabetic subjects and very low in early-onset diabetics and control subjects had intermediate levels. CMPF is associated with pancreatic function. This metabolite causes β-islet cell dysfunction when elevated [26, 27]; CMPF is part of the fatty acid and decarboxylase metabolism pathway. Here, the elevation in CMPF is restricted to late-onset disease compared to early-onset disease, where the levels are actually suppressed in early-onset diabetics compared to control populations (data not shown). This pancreas-related metabolite was the exception between early- and late-onset subjects since in all other six cases the early-onset subject demonstrated the more pronounced defect.

Is there evidence to support the hypothesis that intrinsic pancreas defects unrelated to the immune system contribute to a broader etiologic basis of diabetes, perhaps related to the target organ? Developmental biology has long been ignored in the etiology of autoimmune diseases [28, 29]. In the NOD mouse, there is both support for direct T-cell-driven autoimmunity and secondary organ failure from intrinsic developmental defects. Using NOD-scid mice without an immune system, NOD structural defects related to organogenesis can be observed in the pancreas and salivary glands from birth onward and in other organs. The structurally defective organs share a common developmentally related origin: Hox11-expressing progenitor cells during fetal development [29]. Hox11-derived organs such as the cochlea/inner ear are related to Hox11 developmental biology, as are the sensory portions of the tongue. NOD mice fail to form an inner ear and are born deaf; they also have malformed sensory end organs of the tongue [28]. The human evidence provided here by metabolomics offers additional support for the possibility that intrinsic pancreas developmental defects could contribute, at least in early-onset human diabetes, to more rapid end-organ failure as has been shown in the NOD mouse.

In conclusion, there is supporting evidence from both autoimmune mice and humans that primary, not secondary, additional pancreas dysfunction in diabetes could be driven by developmental biology defects and that associated organs can also fail even without a lymphocyte influence.

5. Implications for therapy

What are the therapeutic implications of the pathophysiological differences underlying early- and late-onset diabetes? For early-onset diabetics, their rapid deficiency in autoreactive T-cells suggests that they are unlikely to respond to immunotherapy aimed at abolishing the autoimmune response if the therapy is started very long after the disease onset. Conversely, for late-onset diabetics, immunotherapies are likely to be effective longer because the patients still have a vigorous autoimmune response and in many cases pancreatic insulin secretion that could be reserved.

The first hint that immunotherapies may be preferentially effective for late-onset diabetes came from a phase I, proof-of-concept clinical trial, published by our laboratory in 2012. It was found that the immunotherapy bacillus Calmette-Guérin (BCG) transiently dampens autoimmunity by selective targeting for death autoreactive T-cells and inducing the beneficial T-regulatory T-cells. With BCG, patients with long-standing disease (mean duration of 15.3 years) fleetingly produced higher levels of C-peptide, showed increases in dead autoreactive T-cells, and produced more T-regulatory cells (Tregs) that suppress autoimmunity. When all weekly blood sera were analyzed by an ultrasensitive assay at the end of the trial, all BCG recipients (as well as placebo controls) were found to have low yet detectable C-peptide secretion.

BCG's apparent efficacy in type 1 diabetes stems from its induction of endogenous tumor necrosis factor (TNF)-α [30], which, in turn, selectively kills CD8+, but not CD4+, autoreactive T-cells in type 1 diabetics and other autoimmune diseases [31]. TNF is also known to expand T-regulatory T-cells as well. TNF itself is not a suitable exogenous immunotherapy because of its high toxicity, which is largely due to widespread expression of the TNF receptor 1 [32]. The TNF inducer BCG is a safer alternative to direct administration of TNF.

BCG is also advantageous because of its FDA approval, low cost, and its 100-year track record of safety as a tuberculosis vaccine and 40-year track record of safety as a treatment for bladder cancer. The BCG trial was among the first immunotherapy clinical trials to include long-standing diabetic subjects, as most if not all of immunotherapy trials over the past 20 years have excluded all but new-onset patients under the now erroneous assumption that β-islets are not salvageable.

A phase II clinical trial of BCG is now in progress, using more frequent doses, a larger group of subjects ($n = 150$), and a 5-year follow-up. The primary objective of this randomized, placebo-controlled double-blind trial is to determine the dose and timing of BCG administration

http://dx.doi.org/10.5772/65598

necessary to trigger a significant improvement in HbA1c values. One of the inclusion criteria is that subjects have fasting or stimulated C-peptide levels between 5 and 200 pmol/L, because these levels are indicative of remaining pancreatic islet function. With the additional criteria that these subjects also must be adults (greater than age 18), the majority of the subjects will also be late-onset subjects.

Two other recent immunotherapy clinical trials in type 1 diabetes, using abatacept and teplizumab, have had disappointing results [33, 34]. One reason postulated to be behind the lackluster results was the heterogeneity of type 1 diabetics, including age of onset [35]. We agree that early- versus late-onset might have been one important source of disease heterogeneity that hampered the trials' success. The results of our BCG trial and the data we have presented here on C-peptide persistence and age of onset suggest that immunotherapy clinical trials no longer exclude all but new-onset cases.

In conclusion, the data that we report here reveal that early- and late-onset diabetics differ in terms of C-peptide production, autoreactive T-cell levels, and metabolites. Taken together, the data suggests that therapies aimed at immune defects are likely to have greater efficacy in late-onset diabetes, whereas therapies aimed at immune defects and β-islet preservation are likely to have greater efficacy in early-onset diabetes.

Acknowledgements

We are grateful for the technical support over the nearly 6 years of this study from Dr. Douglas Burger, Peter Reinhold III, and Sophie L. Washer.

Abbreviations

pMHC-I multimers peptide-major histocompatibility complex class I multimers

AOO age of onset

ER endoplasmic reticulum

T1D type 1 diabetes

Author details

Willem M. Kühtreiber, Miriam Davis and Denise L. Faustman*

*Address all correspondence to: faustman@helix.mgh.harvard.edu

Immunobiology Laboratory, Massachusetts General Hospital, Harvard Medical School, Boston, MA, USA

References

[1] Wang L, Lovejoy NF, Faustman DL. Persistence of prolonged C-peptide production in type 1 diabetes as measured with an ultrasensitive C-peptide assay. Diabetes Care. 2012;35:465–70. DOI:10.2337/dc11-1236.

[2] American Diabetes A. Standards of medical care in diabetes—2014. Diabetes Care. 2014;37 Suppl. 1:S14–80. DOI:10.2337/dc14-S014.

[3] Jones AG, Hattersley AT. The clinical utility of C-peptide measurement in the care of patients with diabetes. Diabetic Medicine: A Journal of the British Diabetic Association. 2013;30:803–17. DOI:10.1111/dme.12159.

[4] Oram RA, Jones AG, Besser RE, Knight BA, Shields BM, Brown RJ, et al. The majority of patients with long-duration type 1 diabetes are insulin microsecretors and have functioning beta cells. Diabetologia. 2014;57:187–91. DOI:10.1007/s00125-013-3067-x.

[5] McGee P, Steffes M, Nowicki M, Bayless M, Gubitosi-Klug R, Cleary P, et al. Insulin secretion measured by stimulated C-peptide in long-established type 1 diabetes in the diabetes control and complications trial (DCCT)/epidemiology of diabetes interventions and complications (EDIC) cohort: a pilot study. Diabetic Medicine: A Journal of the British Diabetic Association. 2014;31:1264–8. DOI:10.1111/dme.12504.

[6] Barker A, Lauria A, Schloot N, Hosszufalusi N, Ludvigsson J, Mathieu C, et al. Age-dependent decline of beta-cell function in type 1 diabetes after diagnosis: a multi-centre longitudinal study. Diabetes, Obesity & Metabolism. 2014;16:262–7. DOI:10.1111/dom.12216.

[7] Kuhtreiber WM, Washer SL, Hsu E, Zhao M, Reinhold P, 3rd, Burger D, et al. Low levels of C-peptide have clinical significance for established type 1 diabetes. Diabetic Medicine: A Journal of the British Diabetic Association. 2015;32:1346-53. DOI:10.1111/dme.12850.

[8] Davis AK, DuBose SN, Haller MJ, Miller KM, DiMeglio LA, Bethin KE, et al. Prevalence of detectable C-peptide according to age at diagnosis and duration of type 1 diabetes. Diabetes Care. 2015;38:476–81. DOI:10.2337/dc14-1952.

[9] Oram RA, McDonald TJ, Shields BM, Hudson MM, Shepherd MH, Hammersley S, et al. Most people with long-duration type 1 diabetes in a large population-based study are insulin microsecretors. Diabetes Care. 2015;38:323–8. DOI:10.2337/dc14-0871.

[10] Effect of intensive therapy on residual beta-cell function in patients with type 1 diabetes in the diabetes control and complications trial. A randomized, controlled trial. The diabetes control and complications trial research group. Annals of Internal Medicine. 1998;128:517–23.

[11] Steffes MW, Sibley S, Jackson M, Thomas W. Beta-cell function and the development of diabetes-related complications in the diabetes control and complications trial. Diabetes Care. 2003;26:832–6.

[12] Lachin JM, McGee P, Palmer JP, Group DER. Impact of C-peptide preservation on metabolic and clinical outcomes in the diabetes control and complications trial. Diabetes. 2014;63:739–48. DOI:10.2337/db13-0881.

[13] Milburn MV, Lawton KA. Application of metabolomics to diagnosis of insulin resistance. Annual Review of Medicine 2013;64:291–305. DOI:10.1146/annurev-med-061511-134747.

[14] Kosanam H, Thai K, Zhang Y, Advani A, Connelly KA, Diamandis EP, et al. Diabetes induces lysine acetylation of intermediary metabolism enzymes in the kidney. Diabetes. 2014;63:2432–9. DOI:10.2337/db12-1770.

[15] Kato T, Shimano H, Yamamoto T, Ishikawa M, Kumadaki S, Matsuzaka T, et al. Palmitate impairs and eicosapentaenoate restores insulin secretion through regulation of SREBP-1c in pancreatic islets. Diabetes. 2008;57:2382–92. DOI:10.2337/db06-1806.

[16] Shimano H, Amemiya-Kudo M, Takahashi A, Kato T, Ishikawa M, Yamada N. Sterol regulatory element-binding protein-1c and pancreatic beta-cell dysfunction. Diabetes, Obesity & Metabolism. 2007;9 Suppl. 2:133–9. DOI:10.1111/j.1463-1326.2007.00779.x.

[17] Wikoff WR, Anfora AT, Liu J, Schultz PG, Lesley SA, Peters EC, et al. Metabolomics analysis reveals large effects of gut microflora on mammalian blood metabolites. Proceedings of the National Academy of Sciences of the United States of America. 2009;106:3698–703. DOI:10.1073/pnas.0812874106.

[18] Riepl RL, Reichardt B, Rauscher J, Tzavella K, Teufel J, Lehnert P. Mediators of exocrine pancreatic secretion induced by intraduodenal application of bile and taurodeoxycholate in man. European Journal of Medical Research 1997;2:23–9.

[19] Williams AJ, Thrower SL, Sequeiros IM, Ward A, Bickerton AS, Triay JM, et al. Pancreatic volume is reduced in adult patients with recently diagnosed type 1 diabetes. The Journal of Clinical Endocrinology and Metabolism. 2012;97:E2109–13. DOI:10.1210/jc.2012-1815.

[20] Seghieri G, Gironi A, Niccolai M, Mammini P, Alviggi L, De Giorgio LA, et al. Serum spermidine oxidase activity in patients with insulin-dependent diabetes mellitus and microvascular complications. Acta Diabetologia Latina 1990;27:303–8.

[21] Welsh N A role for polyamines in glucose-stimulated insulin-gene expression. The Biochemical Journal. 1990;271:393–7.

[22] Welsh N, Sjoholm A. Polyamines and insulin production in isolated mouse pancreatic islets. The Biochemical Journal. 1988;252:701–7.

[23] Sjoholm A, Arkhammar P, Berggren PO, Andersson A. Polyamines in pancreatic islets of obese-hyperglycemic (ob/ob) mice of different ages. American Journal of Physiology-Cell Physiology. 2001;280:C317–23.

[24] Pichiah PB, Sankarganesh A, Kalaiselvi S, Indirani K, Kamalakkannan S, SankarGanesh D, et al. Adriamycin induced spermatogenesis defect is due to the reduction in epididymal adipose tissue mass: a possible hypothesis. Medical Hypotheses. 2012;78:218–20. DOI:10.1016/j.mehy.2011.10.027.

[25] Winegrad AI, Burden CL. Hyperactivity of the glucuronic acid pathway in diabetes mellitus. Transactions of the Association of American Physicians. 1965;78:158–73.

[26] Nolan CJ. Lipotoxicity, beta cell dysfunction, and gestational diabetes. Cell Metabolism. 2014;19:553–4. DOI: 10.1016/j.cmet.2014.03.020.

[27] Prentice KJ, Luu L, Allister EM, Liu Y, Jun LS, Sloop KW, et al. The furan fatty acid metabolite CMPF is elevated in diabetes and induces beta cell dysfunction. Cell Metabolism. 2014;19:653–66. DOI:10.1016/j.cmet.2014.03.008.

[28] Lonyai A, Kodama S, Burger D, Davis M, Faustman DL. The promise of Hox11+ stem cells of the spleen for treating autoimmune diseases. Hormone and Metabolic Research. 2008;40:137–46.

[29] Lonyai A, Kodama S, Burger D, Faustman DL. Fetal Hox11 expression patterns predict defective target organs: a novel link between developmental biology and autoimmunity. Immunology and Cell Biology. 2008;86:301–9.

[30] Bohle A, Nowc C, Ulmer AJ, Musehold J, Gerdes J, Hofstetter AG, et al. Detection of urinary TNF, IL 1, and IL 2 after local BCG immunotherapy for bladder carcinoma. Cytokine. 1990;2:175–81.

[31] Ban L, Zhang J, Wang L, Kuhtreiber W, Burger D, Faustman DL. Selective death of autoreactive T cells in human diabetes by TNF or TNF receptor 2 agonism. Proceedings of the National Academy of Sciences of the United States of America. 2008;105:13644–9.

[32] Hieber U, Heim ME. Tumor necrosis factor for the treatment of malignancies. Oncology. 1994;51:142–53.

[33] Orban T, Bundy B, Becker DJ, DiMeglio LA, Gitelman SE, Goland R, et al. Co-stimulation modulation with abatacept in patients with recent-onset type 1 diabetes: a randomised, double-blind, placebo-controlled trial. Lancet. 2011;378:412–9. DOI: 10.1016/S0140-6736(11)60886-6.

[34] Sherry N, Hagopian W, Ludvigsson J, Jain SM, Wahlen J, Ferry RJ, Jr., et al. Teplizumab for treatment of type 1 diabetes (Protégé study): 1-year results from a randomised, placebo-controlled trial. Lancet. 2011;378:487–97. DOI:10.1016/S0140-6736(11)60931-8.

[35] Pozzilli P Type 1 diabetes mellitus in 2011: heterogeneity of T1DM raises questions for therapy. Nature Reviews Endocrinology. 2012;8:78–80. DOI:10.1038/nrendo.2011.228.

[36] Tirupathi Pichiah PB, Suriyakalaa U, Kamalakkannan S, Kokilavani P, Kalaiselvi S, SankarGanesh D, Gowri J, Archunan G, Cha YS, Achiraman S. Spermidine may decrease ER stress in pancreatic beta cells and may reduce apoptosis via activating AMPK dependent autophagy pathway. Med Hypotheses. 2011;77:677–9. doi: 10.1016/j.mehy.2011.07.014.

Chapter 4

IFN-γ versus IL-17: A Battle During Cardiac Autoimmunity Evolution

Eleonora Kurtenbach and Camila Guerra Martinez

Additional information is available at the end of the chapter

http://dx.doi.org/10.5772/66986

Abstract

Cardiovascular diseases are the leading global cause of death. Cardiomyopathies are the most prevalent forms of heart failure diseases currently. They may have genetic or environmental etiology, and the development of an autoimmune process is essential for the progression of the disease. During an autoimmune response, there is the breakdown of self-tolerance and generation of a T-lymphocytes-mediated cellular autoimmune response and B-lymphocytes-mediated humoral autoimmune response. Lymphocytes perpetuate the autoimmune response throughout the release of cytokines, expansion of autoreactive clones, and attenuation of regulatory mechanisms. Increasing evidences indicate that interferon (IFN)-γ and interleukin (IL)-17 participate during autoimmune disorders development. The use of autoimmune cardiomyopathy models revealed antagonistic functions for both cytokines during the evolution of autoimmune cardiomyopathy: while enhanced IFN-γ levels are associated to a lower disease severity, the levels of IL-17 are inversely correlated to a favorable prognosis. More precisely, recent findings indicate that the IFN-γ/IL-17 ratio in combination with other cytokine levels dictates heart's autoimmunity development and dilatation. In this chapter, we discuss the role played by the autoimmune response in the development of cardiomyopathy. We also discuss some immune mechanisms focused on IFN-γ and IL-17's ability to induce and perpetuate cardiac autoimmunity.

Keywords: autoimmunity, cardiomyopathy, IL-17, IFN-γ and immunological response

1. Introduction

Cardiovascular diseases are responsible for over 17 million deaths per year worldwide, representing the leading cause of deaths globally (WHO 2015—http://www.who.int). Among the main disorders that directly affect the heart and/or circulatory system, there are the coronary heart diseases, cerebrovascular accident, hypertension, peripheral arterial diseases, congenital heart diseases, and heart failure [1]. Currently, cardiomyopathies are the most prevalent form of heart failure [2].

About 30% of cardiomyopathies have genetic origins, most of them are autosomal dominant, but there are also cases of X-linked-recessive inheritance and even mitochondrial DNA mutations. In 2015, more than 110 nuclear and 24 mitochondrial genes were correlated with cardiomyopathies [3–5]. Cardiomyopathy patients showed enhanced expression of the mutated genes *TTN* (titin, 27%), *LLMNA* (laminin A/C, 6%), *MYBPC* (myosin-binding protein C, 3%), *TNNT2* (cardiac troponin C, 3%), *MYH6* (myosin heavy chain 6, 3%), and *SCN5A* (sodium channel voltage-dependent-α5, 3%) [6–8]. In addition to the classic cases of sarcomeric protein mutations, an association between single nucleotide polymorphisms (SNPs) and predisposition to cardiomyopathies in some specific populations has also been reported. These SNPs were mainly observed in genes related to the immune response, such as CTLA-4 (cytotoxic T-lymphocyte antigen-4), IL-6 (interleukin-6), TNF-α (tumor necrosis factor alpha), and HLA (human leukocyte antigen) [9, 10].

Cardiomyopathy can also be induced by excessive alcohol consumption, poisoning by heavy metals or medications (e.g., doxorubicin), metabolic abnormalities, and microbial infections (**Figure 1**) [11]. Among the non-infectious etiologies, alcohol consumption is probably the main cause of cardiomyopathy in the Occidental world [10, 12, 13]. Viral infections are the most common form of microbial-mediated cardiomyopathy in Europe and North America [14]. Analysis of patient biopsies revealed that coxsackie B3 virus infection is the leading cause of cardiomyopathy, followed by parvovirus B19, enterovirus, adenovirus, human herpes virus 6, and HIV infection [15, 16].

In Latin America, Chagas′ cardiomyopathy is one of the most common forms of morbidity and mortality in *Trypanosoma cruzi*-infected people, now estimated in the order of 5.7 million people. Approximately one-third of these patients will develop a dilated chronic form of heart failure associated to a worst clinical prognosis [16, 17]

During the development of cardiomyopathy, these genetic or environmental conditions are considered initiators that cause local damage. The disease progression will activate immune response mechanisms, which may lead to the clearance of the infectious agent and/or the defective cardiomyocytes. However, this initial trigger can also activate an immune status that modulates disease progression to a chronic state of cardiomyopathy **(Figure 1)**. The literature suggests that the development of autoimmune processes is the key element in the progression of cardiomyopathy regardless of its etiological origin [11, 18]. Nonetheless, the specific role of the complex immune system response in the induction of cardiac autoimmunity and perpetuation of cardiomyopathy is poorly understood. Recent findings that shed some light in the immune mechanisms of cardiomyopathy induction will be described below.

http://dx.doi.org/10.5772/66986

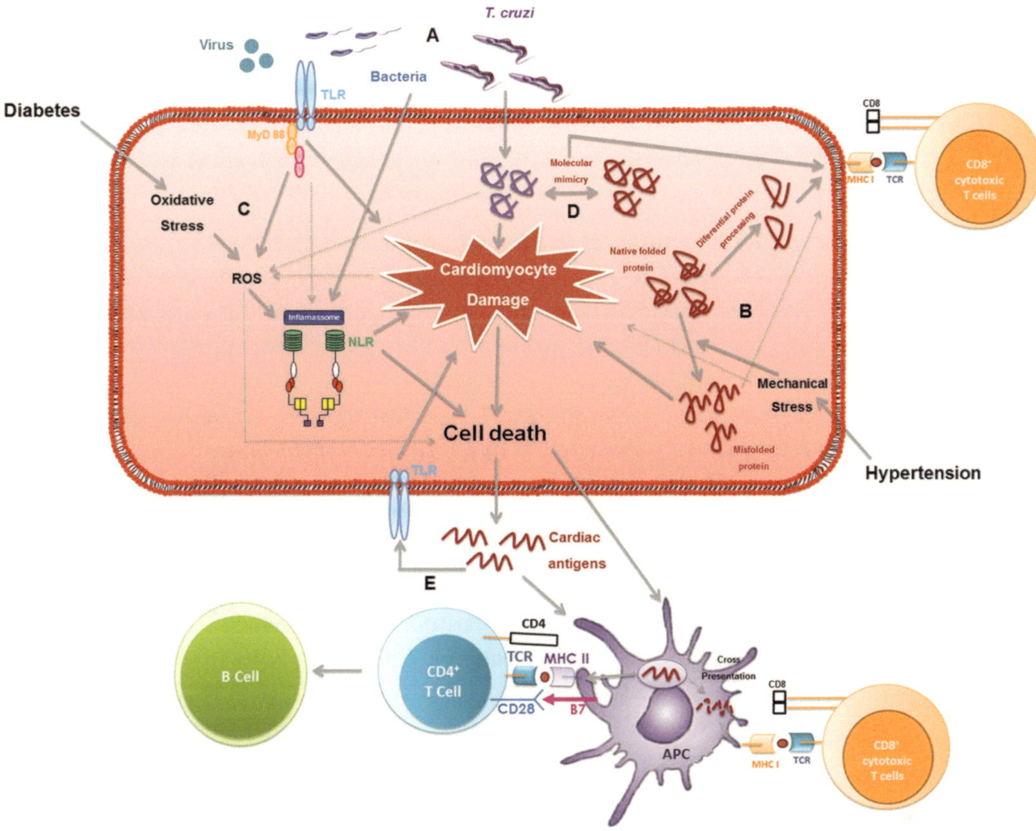

Figure 1. Proposed mechanisms in the development of cardiac autoimmunity. Infection caused by virus, bacteria, protozoa, and other stimuli (A) are recognized by receptors of the innate response, such as TLR and NLRs, leading to cardiomyocytes damage and death. During this process, the assembly of a multiprotein complex known as inflammasome may occur, responsible for secretion of cytokines and the amplification of an autoimmunity cascade. Also, diseases as diabetes and hypertension may activate oxidative and mechanical stress responses, respectively (B and C). These can lead to a redox imbalance and a change in protein processing, amplifying the heart damage. Proteins from infectious agents may exhibit similarity with host proteins, a process known as molecular mimicry (D). All these processes jointly or separately will provoke the exposure of cardiac antigens via MHC I by cardiomyocytes or via MHC II by antigen-presenting cells (APCs) after cardiac antigens or apoptotic cardiomyocytes phagocytosis. These processes will stimulate B-cells, CD4⁺ and CD8⁺ T-cells to mount humoral and cellular autoimmune responses. Besides, cardiac antigens can stimulate additional damages via TLR activation (E), as positive feedback. Gray continuous arrows represent mechanisms described in this review while gray dashed arrows not.

2. Development of cardiac autoimmunity

Cardiomyocyte cellular damage may be induced by infection with pathogens, endogenous stress from mechanical or oxidative traumas, or from mutated proteins (**Figure 1A–C**) [19–22]. These insults promote activation of the innate immune response through pattern recognition receptors (PRRs), such as Toll-like receptors (TLRs) and Nod-like receptors (NLRs). PRRs are expressed in immune cells, such as macrophages, dendritic cells and lymphocytes, cardiac fibroblasts, and cardiomyocytes (**Figure 1**) [23–26]. Activation of heart receptors such as TLR2, TLR4, and TLR5 induces the expression of IL-6, MIP-2 (macrophage inflammatory protein 2), KC (CXCL 1 – homolog of human IL-8), and ICAM-1 (intercellular adhesion molecule-1), and is associated with a decrease in cardiomyocyte contractility [26, 27]. The absence of host immunity receptors or associated pathway components inhibits the development of cardiomyopathies, as observed using an autoimmune animal model in mice depleted for TLR-7$^{-/-}$, TLR-9$^{-/-}$, and MyD88$^{-/-}$ [28].

The listed factors may cause a chronic condition and lead to the activation of cell death mechanisms by apoptosis or necrosis [29–31]. Apoptotic cardiomyocytes are processed by antigen-presenting cells, such as dendritic cells and macrophages, resulting in immune system activation, myocarditis, and production of autoantibodies against heart protein, as anti-myosin antibodies [32, 33]. The death of cardiomyocytes releases autoantigens which are captured by dendritic cells and leads to a "self-aggressive" state through the activation of CD40 and TLR receptors. This dendritic cell-mediated activation mechanism is an important regulator of CD4$^+$ T-cell function [32, 34]. The endocytosed cardiac antigens will be processed and coupled to a molecule of major histocompatibility complex class II (MHC II) and presented via T-cell receptor (TCR) to a CD4$^+$ T-cell **(Figure 1)**. In addition to this initial interaction, the correct activation of the CD4$^+$ T-cell requires a second positive signal that is stimulated by costimulatory molecules such as CD28 and B7 (CD80 and CD86). However, inhibitory signals, such as mediated by CTLA4 molecules, are capable of competing with CD28 for binding to B7, reducing T-cell expansion and production of cytokines [35]. T-cells that do not express the CTLA4-B7-inhibitory signal exhibit an unregulated proliferation of lymphocytes in the heart, which can lead to a severe damage of myocardium, and the development of cardiomyopathies [36, 37]. Cardiomyopathy patients present higher levels of CTLA4 SNP (+49A>G; Thr17Ala), which lead to a loss of function of CTLA4, than healthy subjects (14.7% vs. 7.4%, $p = 0.005$) [38]. Therefore, the correct activation of CD4$^+$ T-cells in cardiac autoimmunity is mediated by (1) antigen-presenting cells that phagocytosed death cardiomyocytes or cardiac autoantigens and (2) a second co-stimulatory signal mediated by B7 **(Figure 1)**. In addition to antigen-presenting cells, other cell types of non-hematopoietic lineage can also present antigens to CD4$^+$ T-cells via MHC II under inflammatory stimuli [39]. It has been shown in patients and in rodent models that the MHC II expression by non-hematopoietic cells, in particular endothelial cells, contributes to the development of cardiomyopathy [40, 41]. Mice developed lower cardiac commitment when they did not express MHC II in endothelial cells [41]. Finally, properly activated CD4$^+$ T-cells are able to activate B-lymphocytes to produce and secrete antibodies against cardiac antigens. The role of B-cells during the development of heart disease has been extensively studied [42]. The absence of programmed cell death protein-1 (PD-1), a key factor in the differentiation of B cells, can lead to the development of a severe form of dilated cardiomyopathy, with high levels of IgG that specifically binds to cardiomyocytes and induce apoptosis [43, 44]. Depletion of these B-cells recovers the heart failure phenotype in mice [42]. The production and release of autoantibodies is dependent of B-cell differentiation to plasma cells. During this process, there is a decrease in CD19 expression and maintenance of high levels of CD138 and transcription factor Blimp-1 [45]. The expression of these two factors is dependent of high levels of IL-17 and activation of autophagy. After this differentiation, it is possible to observe high titers of anti-myosin antibodies in BALB/c mice

http://dx.doi.org/10.5772/66986

immunized with α-myosin heavy chain peptide (α-Myhc), particularly IgG2a and IgG2b subtypes, and the development of some cardiac impairment characteristics, such as the increase in the ratio of heart and body weight [46]. These antibodies can recognize and bind to specific cardiac antigens and deposited into the myocardium [47]. A wide range of evidence suggests that these autoantibodies directly affect cardiac function and physiology [48].

In addition to the response mediated by $CD4^+$ T- and B-cells, $CD8^+$ T-cytotoxic lymphocytes may be activated through the recognition of conjugated epitopes on MHC I. Damage induced by pathogen infection or cell stress mechanisms can alter intracellular protein processing resulting in misfolding, which will expose it to MHC I molecules. This will expose self-epitopes to autoreactive $CD8^+$ T-cells (**Figure 1A**, **B** and **D**) [13]. Also, molecular mimicry may occur between pathogens and heart proteins (**Figure 1B** and **D**) [49]. This latter mechanism is well described in Chagas' patients where antibodies against the B13 *T. cruzi* protein can also recognize cardiac α-Myhc (**Figure 1D**) [50]. This step via MHC I will promote the release of cytotoxic agents, such as perforin and granzyme B by $CD8^+$ T-cells that could promote cardiomyocytes apoptosis and can amplify the release of cardiac antigens [51]. Throughout the modulation of immune system, lymphocytes will release cytokines that will expand autoreactive clones propagating the autoimmune response [11]. The autoimmune process formed by humoral and cellular responses can amplify the cardiac damage through the secretion of autoantibodies, cytokines, and other immune factors, despite initial stimuli.

Analysis of cardiomyopathy patients revealed the presence of autoantibodies against self-myocardial protein in up to 80% of the patients [52], indicating that autoimmunity is a central element for cardiomyopathy development. Evidence indicates that these autoantibodies affect the heart rather than other organs. Serum or IgG purified from these patients can induce negative inotropic effects on the heart of chicken embryos [53] and decrease heart contraction, the calcium transport [54, 55], and the diastolic relaxation in mice [48, 56]. The transference of IgG purified from patients serum with cardiac dysfunction to healthy mice induced significant necrosis in cardiomyocytes and mediated inflammatory effects with the aid of immune cells [57]. The characterization of these antibodies started in the 1980s and continues until today. Some of these antigens are listed in **Table 1** [58–69]. Most of produced autoantibodies directly recognize one specific cardiac antigen. But it has been demonstrated in rats that anti-myosin antibodies are capable to recognize the β1-adrenergic receptor and promotes their activation [70].

As briefly discussed above, the mechanisms that trigger the development of autoimmune cardiomyopathy are orchestrated by humoral and cellular responses. Immune cells such as granulocytes, monocytes, T-cells, B-cells, and mast cells infiltrate into the heart and promote the secretion of the cytokines, IL-17, -6, -1, -10, -12, IFN-γ, TGF-β, TNF-α, and chemokines that will generate an amplification loop, recruiting new inflammatory cells to the heart [71–77]. However, the precise elucidation of this complex immune response mechanism remains unclear due to the difficulty to determine the precise order that immune cells infiltrate the heart [78–80]. Once activated, this cellular response will undergo both beneficial and harmful effects as the disease progresses.

Data obtained in experimental autoimmune cardiomyopathy models using immunization with α-Myhc showed a predominance of $CD4^+$ T-cell response [41, 77, 78, 81]. The transfer

Class of cardiac protein	Protein	First citation
G protein–coupled receptors	β1 adrenergic receptor	Limas et al., [58]
	2 muscarinic receptor	Fu et al., [59]
Mitochondrial	M7 antigen	Klein et al. [60]
	Adenine nucleotide translocase (ANT)	Schultheiss et al. [61]
Structural	α-myosin heavy chain (MyHC)	Neu et al. [62]
	Troponin I	Okazaki et al. [63]
	Laminin	Wolff et al. [64]
	Myosin-binding protein-C	Müller et al. [65]
	Dystrophin	Müller et al. [65]
Others	Na-K ATPase	Baba et al. [66]
	Hsp-60	Latif et al. [67]
	Proteasome 20 S	Voigt et al. [68]
	Calreticulin	Sánchez et al. [69]
	RNA-binding protein 20	Müller et al. [65]

Table 1. Cardiac antigens characterized in autoimmune cardiomyopathies.

of $CD4^+$ T-cells from mouse spleen that produced anti-myosin antibodies and developed cardiomyopathy mimics the disease in severe combined immunodeficiency (SCID) mice. On the contrary, $CD8^+$ T-cell transference did not induce changes [32, 82]. Moreover, the depletion of $CD4^+$ T-cells or treatment with anti-CD4 antibody prevents acute myocarditis with a decrease in the antibodies production and heart size [18, 83], confirming a prominent $CD4^+$ T-cell role in this autoimmune cardiomyopathy model.

$CD4^+$ T-lymphocytes can be biased to different profiles: Th1, Th2, Th17, Th9, Th22, follicular T (Tfh cells), and induced regulatory T (Treg cells) cells, each of which has a specialized function and is adapted to suppress a specific class of injuries or counteract the excessive activation of the immune system [84]. For autoimmune cardiomyopathy, the involvement of Th1, Th2, and Th17 cells has been characterized. The most relevant studies in this area are focused on Th1 and Th17 responses and their respective cytokines [32, 71–73, 76, 85–88].

3. IL-17 *versus* IFN-γ

Early studies using immunohistochemical assays identified the presence of cells producing mainly TNF-α and IL-1 in heart [89, 90]. In the early 2000 era, novel cytokines were identified in cardiomyopathic animal as IL-2 and IL-1-β [91]. In 2006, the first evidence of the IL-17 participation in autoimmune cardiomyopathy [76] was described.

In the last decade, Th17 cells have been extensively characterized in various autoimmune diseases [92, 93], including autoimmune cardiomyopathy [3, 80, 94]. Th17 $CD4^+$ T-cells have been named after the discovery of their classical cytokine, IL-17A, but they also produce other effector cytokines including IL-17F, IL-22, and granulocyte macrophage-colony-stimulating factor (GM-CSF) [95]. Additionally, IL-17 may also be secreted by other cell types as Th17 $CD8^+$ T-cells (Tc17), γδ T-cells (mainly in the skin and intestine), mucosal-associated invariant T-cells (MAIT), among other resident T-cells in different tissues [96, 97]. The polarization of $CD4^+$ T-cells to Th17 profile initially requires the presence of TGF-β. This cytokine induces the expression of ROR-γt (RAR-related orphan receptor-γt) and FoxP3 (Forkhead box P3) transcriptional factors [98]. The co-expression of these two factors allows the physical connection between FoxP3 and ROR-γt inhibiting their differentiation to Th17. In the presence of IL-6, STAT3 is activated and interrupts the inhibition induced by FoxP3, resulting in the expression of IL-23 receptor and initiating the differentiation to Th17. Nevertheless, in the absence of IL-6, the inhibition of ROR-γt induced by FoxP3 will favor the development and expansion of Treg cells [99]. Beyond IL-6, IL-1-β is also capable of inhibiting FoxP3, generating an amplification loop [100, 101]. This cytokine polarization is very well characterized to $CD4^+$ T-cells, but also appear to be responsible for differentiation of $CD8^+$ T-cells to Tc17 profile [102, 103]. Recently, it was demonstrated that the differentiation of $CD8^+$ T for IL-17 producing $CD8^+$ T-cells is also dependent on the inhibition of Blimp-1 and T-bet [104]. Today, it is well accepted that the release of cytokines required for this process of differentiation, such as IL-6, IL-12, TNF-α, and IL-23 by antigen-presenting cells, such as dendritic cells and $CD14^+$ monocyte, is induced by the recognition of cardiac autoantigens by TLR and by the presence of GM-CSF [105, 106]. As described, IL-6 and IL-23 will induce the differentiation of T helper (Th) cells to Th17 profile, where the release of IL-17 and more GM-CSF occurs, forming a positive feedback [88, 94].

Several works published in the last 10 years, using animal models and patients with cardiomyopathy, tried to establish IL-17 as a cytokine inducer of autoimmune cardiomyopathy. IL-17 was described as an important factor responsible for cardiac remodeling, fibrosis, and many other effects in the heart [72, 78, 86, 88]. An increase in IL-17 and IFN-γ transcriptional levels in mice that develop experimental autoimmune myocarditis (EAM) induced by subcutaneous inoculation with α-Myhc was observed. In this case, the copy number of IL-17 mRNA was about 20–30 times higher than those to IFN-γ [107].

It has been shown that the presence of IL-17 increases the expression of MMP-1 (matrix metalloproteinase-1), promoting the migration of cardiac fibroblasts *in vitro* and cardiac remodeling *in vivo* [108]. Furthermore, it was shown that Th17 cells and IL-17 were involved in survival, proliferation, and differentiation of B-cells [109]. In this direction, sera of patients with dilated cardiomyopathy showed an increase in IL-17 levels and in the frequency of Th17 cells when compared to health donors [109]. IL-17 neutralization or depletion slowed the development of autoimmune response and reduced the generation of cardiac autoantibodies in EAM myosin model [76, 110]. Also, mice treated with anti-IL-6, which were not capable of promoting the polarization of $CD4^+$ T-cells to Th17 profile, do not develop autoimmune cardiomyopathy [111].

But these facts seem to be true only in the acute phase of the disease. After the establishment of a chronic condition, patients with cardiomyopathy presented lower levels of IL-17 and Th17 cells subtype [112]. So, high IL-17 levels are essential in acute phase of cardiomyopathy and for the progression to the final stage of the disease. But when the cardiomyopathy reaches this final stage, where heart dilatation is found, IL-17 seems not necessary [86, 87]. And even more, the reduction of IL-17 levels after the establishment of cardiac damage did not appear to be beneficial. In fact, mice infected with *T. cruzi* presenting typical functional cardiomyopathy changes, when treated with anti-IL17, developed an acute exacerbation of inflammation and cardiac dysfunction [113]. The absence of IL-17 receptor on infected mice also leads to the development of a fatal cardiomyopathy [114]. Additionally, it was demonstrated that individuals infected with *T. cruzi* who developed severe cardiac dysfunction had lower levels of IL-17 when compared with infected patients presenting moderate symptoms [115]. Recently, a study analyzed IL-17 levels in blood sample of 41 patients with dilated cardiomyopathy, without differentiating the etiology of the disease. They observed an increase in IL-17 levels up to 6 months after the diagnosis, but after 1 year of monitoring, IL-17 levels reduced close to those found in healthy patients, even in the presence of high levels of IL-6 and TGF-β [94]. This association between reduction in IL-17 levels and worse prognosis has also been found in patients who suffered acute myocardial infarction [116]. Finally, our research group recently showed that this relationship between IL-17 late decrease and worse symptoms occurred in heart disease of autoimmune origin. Mice that produce anti-M_2AChR antibodies induced by gene immunization showed dilated cardiomyopathy and an increase in IL-17 production in the heart at 20-week postimmunization; however, with the progression of the disease to a final dilated stage, about 40 weeks after immunization, the IL-17 levels become comparable to the levels produced by the respective control animals [117]. The literature did not present explanations about the mechanisms involved in decreasing IL-17 levels. But IL-17 reduction, after the achievement of the disease, seems to be more harmful than beneficial to the development of cardiomyopathy. Thus, it is crucial to emphasize that the use of anti-IL-17 therapies for heart disease and other autoimmune diseases needs to be employed in a precise time to avoid harmful effects in the patients.

The immune response via Th1 cells and their cytokine marker IFN-γ is also largely related to autoimmune cardiomyopathy. During the innate immune response, IFN-γ is produced by natural killer cells and natural killer T-cells [118], as well as macrophages and dendritic cells [119]. In adaptive immunity, IFN-γ is mainly produced by $CD8^+$ T-cells and Th1 $CD4^+$ T-cells [120, 121]. After TCR stimulation, $CD8^+$ T-cells produce higher levels of IFN-γ than $CD4^+$ T-cells [122]. This is possible due to the interaction between TCR-MHC interaction that occurs between the $CD8^+$ T-cells and MHC I-expressing antigen-presenting cells is sufficient to induce the secretion of IFN-γ and differentiation to a cytotoxic profile, whereas $CD4^+$ T-cells need TCR recognition and a series of other stimuli [120]. IFN-γ also contributes to the switch process of IgG subclass in B-cells to a more pathogenic profile (IgG2a and IgG3 subclasses), activation of the complement system, inflammation, and tissue damage [123, 124]. But the IFN-γ expression is not static and confined to these classic subtype cells described above. Th17 cells can also produce IFN-γ concomitantly with IL-17 and even can become an exclusive IFN-γ producer [125, 126].

http://dx.doi.org/10.5772/66986

IFN-γ is an indicator of pathogenicity for autoimmune diseases [127], but its role in cardiomyopathies is still controversial [128] and it appears to be more protective than inducer of disease [76, 85, 129–131]. For instance, mice treated with anti-IFN-γ antibodies or genetic deleted for T-bet, IFN-γ, or IFN-γR presented an exacerbated inflammatory infiltrates and increased heart size and its cavities [71–73, 76, 85, 130]. One of the possible protective mechanisms mediated by IFN-γ involves the inhibition of autoreactive T-cell proliferation through the induction of nitric oxide synthase 2 enzyme (NOS2) and nitric oxide (NO) release [77, 132]. Although today this mechanism seems simple, its elucidation was very contradictory and troubled for some years. Initially, IL12Rβ1, one of the IL-12 receptor subunits, knockout mice were used for the study of participation of the IFN-γ in autoimmune cardiomyopathy. The inhibition of this classically Th1-polarizing pathway decreased the development of autoimmune cardiomyopathy in knockout mice, indicating the pathogenicity of Th1 cells [85]. However, as already mentioned, the IFN-$\gamma^{-/-}$ and IFN-$\gamma R^{-/-}$ mice showed an exaggerated and lethal disease [72, 73], an apparent contradictory result. This impasse was resolved when it was shown that β1 subunit of the receptor for IL-12 was shared with the IL-23 receptor, inducer of Th17 response [110]. Despite all this characterization of IFN-γ-protective role, it is unclear which mechanisms are activated during this process. It is known that high levels of IFN-γ induce the production of NO by NOS2 with consequently inhibition of $CD4^+$ T-cells autoreactive proliferation [77]. HL-1 cell line and primary cardiomyocytes treated with IFN-γ showed an activation of absent in melanoma 2 (AIM-2), an intracellular receptor of the PRRs family, which reduces IL-6, IP-10 (inducible protein 10, CXCL10), and TNF-α transcription in cardiomyocytes and limits inflammation in cardiomyocytes, but not in cardiac fibroblasts [133]. Also, high IFN-γ levels secreted by γδ cells could kill pathogenic $F4/80^+$ macrophages in heart and control cardiac damage [134]. There could be some explanation for how IFN-γ protects mice from the development of autoimmune cardiomyopathy.

Meanwhile, several other studies demonstrated the ability of high IFN-γ levels in inducing myocardial inflammation, interstitial fibrosis, apoptosis, wall thinning, systolic dysfunction, dilatation, and cardiomyopathy [128]. And more recently, it has been shown that IFN-γ has the capacity to induce cardiac damage in autoimmune cardiomyopathy model. High IFN-γ levels were associated with cardiorespiratory commitment, electrical abnormalities, and cardiac dilatation. This situation was more prominent in the absence of purinergic receptor P2X7 [117]. These evidences show that it is not possible to withdraw the IFN-γ participation as a cardiomyopathy inducer.

4. Immune cells' function on autoimmune cardiomyopathy

The entire description and discussion made so far focused mainly on the presence and polarization of $CD4^+$ T-cells; however, as already pointed out, the presence and participation of other immune cells can be decisive in disease severity. In genetically susceptible mouse model, preferably BALB/c, immunization with the α-Myhc in the presence of a strong adjuvant, like complete Freund's adjuvant (CFA), the disease is mediated almost exclusively by $CD4^+$ T-cells. However, it has been recently identified in EAM-induced A/J mice that the

α-Myhc$_{338\text{-}348}$ epitope was the immune dominant for CD8$^+$ response [135]. In this case, they showed antibodies production, cardiomyopathy development, and the presence of inflammatory infiltrate composed of 35% of CD8$^+$ T-cells [135]. As previously mentioned, this infiltration of CD8$^+$ T-cells has a high cytotoxic role as a source of IFN-γ, perforin, and granzyme that will induce irreversible damage to cardiomyocytes [51].

Despite the great importance of T-cells, it is believed that the major cells infiltrating the hearts during the development of cardiomyopathy are monocytes, especially CD11b$^+$ [77]. These cells can differentiate into different profiles ranging from dendritic cells, macrophages, and fibroblasts depending on the immune environment (including cytokines, chemokines, and growth factors) present in the heart [77, 132, 136]. The more severe cardiomyopathy is found when there is the presence of eosinophils in the heart infiltration [131]. It is believed that NK cells control the exacerbated proliferation of eosinophils in the heart through direct induction of apoptosis [137]. The recruitment of eosinophils to the heart can also be controlled by cardiac fibroblasts and F4/80$^+$ macrophages through the release of CCL11 and CCL24 (eotaxin-1 and eotaxin-2), respectively [138].

In the healthy heart, it is possible to find a population of resident macrophages, but the number of these cells can be expanded after the infiltration of new macrophages under some stimulus such as initiators of the autoimmune cardiomyopathy, cited at the beginning of this review (Figure 1). Macrophage infiltration is a well-known step, but it is little studied in cardiomyopathy [139]. These cells can differentiate into various profiles depending on the cytokine present in the medium. Some of these profiles are classically activated, pro-inflammatory M1 macrophages and alternatively activated, anti-inflammatory M2-polarized macrophages, tumor-associated macrophages (TAM), "immature" monocyte-like (GR1/Ly6C$^+$) or "mature" neutrophil-like (GR1/Ly6G$^+$), and suppressor cells derived from myeloid precursor (MDSCs) [79]. The functional properties and secretory profile of macrophages likely promote myocardial health or disease. In some cases, their influence on acute inflammation and chronic fibrosis is well described, and in others, their cardioprotective function seems to be almost indisputable, being proposed as a good source of treatment [140–142]. In models of cardiac autoimmunity, there is a predominance of M2 macrophages, around 70%, which promoted the resolution of the disease in heart tissue after damage. And with the presence of M1 macrophages, there is the expansion of Th17 cells and cardiac dilation [79, 143–145]. Therefore, further studies about the importance and function of macrophages in cardiomyopathies, in particular autoimmune ones, are needed.

5. Conclusion

The findings described in this chapter demonstrate the existence of a precise balance of the immune response, where a complex network of factors creates the conditions for the progression of autoimmune cardiomyopathy and dictates its severity. The combination of present and future knowledge on this line of study can ultimately guide to a possible effective and non-general treatment. However, two factors must be taken into consideration: (1) the correct association between anti-humoral and anti-cytokine therapies and (2) the period where the treatment must be applied.

Therefore, the participation of IFN-γ and IL-17 in the autoimmunity development recalls us a dance instead of an arms race, where a fine temporal and quantitative control of these cytokines can determine the cardiomyopathy evolution.

Acknowledgements

Sources of funding for this work were from the Fundação de Amparo a Pesquisa do Rio de Janeiro – FAPERJ/Temáticos and Instituto Nacional para Pesquisa Translacional em Saúde e Ambiente na Região Amazônica – INPETAM, Conselho Nacional de Desenvolvimento Científico e Tecnológico/ MCT. We thank Dr Pedro Muanis Persechini and Dr Rafael Soares Aquino for review and final formatting of this review. The authors declare that they have no conflicts of interest.

Author details

Eleonora Kurtenbach* and Camila Guerra Martinez

*Address all correspondence to: kurten@biof.ufrj.br

Federal University of Rio de Janeiro, Rio de Janeiro, Brazil

References

[1] BJ Maron, JA Towbin, G Thiene, C Antzelevitch, D Corrado, D Arnett, AJ Moss, CE Seidman, and JB Young. Contemporary definitions and classification of the cardiomyopathies an American heart association scientific statement from the council on clinical cardiology, heart failure and transplantation committee; quality of care and outcomes research and functional genomics and translational biology interdisciplinary working groups; and council on epidemiology and prevention. Circulation. 2006; **113**:1807–1816. DOI: 10.1161/CIRCULATIONAHA.106.174287.

[2] GV Ramani, PA Uber, and MR Mehra. Chronic heart failure: contemporary diagnosis and management. Mayo Clinic Proceedings. 2010; **85**:180–195. DOI: 10.4065/mcp.2009.0494.

[3] NR Rose. Myocarditis: infection versus autoimmunity. Journal of Clinical Immunology. 2009; **29**:730–737. DOI: 10.1007/s10875-009-9339-z.

[4] T Shaw, P Elliott, and WJ McKenna. Dilated cardiomyopathy: a genetically heterogeneous disease. The Lancet. 2002; **360**:654–655. DOI: 10.1016/S0140-6736(02)09879-3.

[5] M Harakalova, G Kummeling, A Sammani, M Linschoten, AF Baas, J van der Smagt, PA Doevendans, JP van Tintelen, D Dooijes, and M Mokry. A systematic analysis of genetic

dilated cardiomyopathy reveals numerous ubiquitously expressed and muscle-specific genes. European Journal of Heart Failure. 2015; **17**:484–493. DOI: 10.1002/ejhf.255.

[6] DS Herman, L Lam, MR Taylor, L Wang, P Teekakirikul, D Christodoulou, L Conner, SR DePalma, B McDonough, and E Sparks. Truncations of titin causing dilated cardiomyopathy. New England Journal of Medicine. 2012; **366**:619–628. DOI: 10.1056/NEJMoa1110186.

[7] RE Hershberger and JD Siegfried. Update 2011: clinical and genetic issues in familial dilated cardiomyopathy. Journal of the American College of Cardiology. 2011; **57**:1641–1649. DOI: 10.1016/j.jacc.2011.01.015.

[8] YM Pinto, PM Elliott, E Arbustini, Y Adler, A Anastasakis, M Böhm, D Duboc, J Gimeno, P de Groote, and M Imazio. Proposal for a revised definition of dilated cardiomyopathy, hypokinetic non-dilated cardiomyopathy, and its implications for clinical practice: a position statement of the ESC working group on myocardial and pericardial diseases. European Heart Journal. 2016; **37**:1850–1858. DOI: 10.1093/eurheartj/ehv727.

[9] J Staab, V Ruppert, S Pankuweit, and T Meyer. Polymorphisms in genes encoding non-sarcomeric proteins and their role in the pathogenesis of dilated cardiomyopathy. Herz. 2012; **37**:836–842. DOI: 10.1007/s00059-012-3698-6.

[10] S Pankuweit, V Ruppert, u Jónsdóttir, H-H Müller, T Meyer, and GCNoH Failure. The HLA class II allele DQB1* 0309 is associated with dilated cardiomyopathy. Gene. 2013; **531**:180–183.

[11] JM Lappé, CM Pelfrey, and WW Tang. Recent insights into the role of autoimmunity in idiopathic dilated cardiomyopathy. Journal of Cardiac Failure. 2008; **14**:521–530. DOI: 10.1016/j.cardfail.2008.02.016.

[12] GM Felker, RE Thompson, JM Hare, RH Hruban, DE Clemetson, DL Howard, KL Baughman, and EK Kasper. Underlying causes and long-term survival in patients with initially unexplained cardiomyopathy. New England Journal of Medicine. 2000; **342**:1077–1084. DOI: 10.1056/NEJM200004133421502.

[13] S Pankuweit, V Ruppert, and B Maisch. Inflammation in dilated cardiomyopathy. Herz. 2004; **29**:788–793. DOI: 10.1007/s00059-004-2626-9.

[14] H Mahrholdt, A Wagner, CC Deluigi, E Kispert, S Hager, G Meinhardt, H Vogelsberg, P Fritz, J Dippon, and C-T Bock. Presentation, patterns of myocardial damage, and clinical course of viral myocarditis. Circulation. 2006; **114**:1581–1590. DOI: 10.1161/CIRCULATIONAHA.105.606509.

[15] U Kühl, M Pauschinger, B Seeberg, D Lassner, M Noutsias, W Poller, and H-P Schultheiss. Viral persistence in the myocardium is associated with progressive cardiac dysfunction. Circulation. 2005; **112**:1965–1970. DOI: 10.1161/CIRCULATIONAHA.105.548156.

[16] T Leslie Jr, A Keren, K Sliwa, A Matsumori, and GA Mensah. The global burden of myocarditis. Global Heart. 2014; **9**:121–129. DOI: 10.1016/j.gheart.2014.01.007.

[17] EA Bocchi, FGM Braga, SMA Ferreira, LEP Rohde, WAd Oliveira, DRd Almeida, MdCV Moreira, RB Bestetti, S Bordignon, and C Azevedo. III Brazilian Guideline for Insufficiency Chronic heart disease. Brazilian Archives of Cardiology. 2009; **93**:3–70. DOI: 10.1590/S0066-782X2009002000001

[18] T Yoshikawa, A Baba, and Y Nagatomo. Autoimmune mechanisms underlying dilated cardiomyopathy. Circulation Journal. 2009; **73**:602–607. DOI: 10.1253/circj.CJ-08-1151.

[19] N Bodyak, PM Kang, M Hiromura, I Sulijoadikusumo, N Horikoshi, K Khrapko, and A Usheva. Gene expression profiling of the aging mouse cardiac myocytes. Nucleic Acids Research. 2002; **30**:3788–3794. DOI: 10.1093/nar/gkf497.

[20] KM Bonney and DM Engman. Chagas heart disease pathogenesis: one mechanism or many? Current Molecular Medicine. 2008; **8**:510–518. DOI: 10.2174/156652408785748004.

[21] Z Cai, L Shen, H Ma, J Yang, D Yang, H Chen, J Wei, Q Lu, DW Wang, and M Xiang. Involvement of endoplasmic reticulum stress-mediated C/EBP homologous protein activation in coxsackievirus B3-induced acute viral myocarditis. Circulation: Heart Failure. 2015; **8**:809–818. DOI: 10.1161/CIRCHEARTFAILURE.114.001244.

[22] G Gao, J Zhang, X Si, J Wong, C Cheung, B McManus, and H Luo. Proteasome inhibition attenuates coxsackievirus-induced myocardial damage in mice. American Journal of Physiology-Heart and Circulatory Physiology. 2008; **295**:H401–H408. DOI: 10.1152/ajpheart.00292.2008.

[23] S Akira, S Uematsu, and O Takeuchi. Pathogen recognition and innate immunity. Cell. 2006; **124**:783–801. DOI: 10.1016/j.cell.2006.02.015.

[24] L Lin and AA Knowlton. Innate immunity and cardiomyocytes in ischemic heart disease. Life Sciences. 2014; **100**:1–8. DOI: 10.1016/j.lfs.2014.01.062.

[25] KL Rock, E Latz, F Ontiveros, and H Kono. The sterile inflammatory response. Annual Review of Immunology. 2010; **28**:321–342. DOI: 10.1146/annurev-immunol-030409-101311.

[26] JH Boyd, S Mathur, Y Wang, RM Bateman, and KR Walley. Toll-like receptor stimulation in cardiomyocytes decreases contractility and initiates an NF-κB dependent inflammatory response. Cardiovascular Research. 2006; **72**:384–393. DOI: 10.1016/j.cardiores.2006.09.011.

[27] C Lipps, JH Nguyen, L Pyttel, TL Lynch, C Liebetrau, G Aleshcheva, S Voss, O Dörr, HM Nef, and H Möllmann. N-terminal fragment of cardiac myosin binding protein-C triggers pro-inflammatory responses in vitro. Journal of Molecular and Cellular Cardiology. 2016; **99**:47–56. DOI: 10.1016/j.yjmcc.2016.09.003.

[28] PP Pagni, S Traub, O Demaria, L Chasson, and L Alexopoulou. Contribution of TLR7 and TLR9 signaling to the susceptibility of MyD88-deficient mice to myocarditis. Autoimmunity. 2010; **43**:275–287. DOI: 10.3109/08916930903509056.

[29] KJ Jensen, FS Garmaroudi, J Zhang, J Lin, S Boroomand, M Zhang, Z Luo, D Yang, H Luo, and BM McManus. An ERK-p38 subnetwork coordinates host cell apoptosis and

necrosis during coxsackievirus B3 infection. Cell Host & Microbe. 2013; **13**:67–76. DOI: 10.1016/j.chom.2012.11.009.

[30] AM Orogo and ÅB Gustafsson. Cell death in the myocardium: my heart won't go on. IUBMB life. 2013; **65**:651–656.

[31] A Piek, R de Boer, and H Silljé. The fibrosis-cell death axis in heart failure. Heart Failure Reviews. 2016; **21**:199–211. DOI: 10.1007/s10741-016-9536-9.

[32] U Eriksson, R Ricci, L Hunziker, MO Kurrer, GY Oudit, TH Watts, I Sonderegger, K Bachmaier, M Kopf, and JM Penninger. Dendritic cell–induced autoimmune heart failure requires cooperation between adaptive and innate immunity. Nature Medicine. 2003; **9**:1484–1490. DOI: 10.1038/nm960

[33] E Wan, X-Y Yeap, S Dehn, RL Terry, ML Novak, S Zhang, S Iwata, X Han, S Homma, and K Drosatos. Enhanced efferocytosis of apoptotic cardiomyocytes through MER tyrosine kinase links acute inflammation resolution to cardiac repair after infarction. Circulation Research. 2013; **113**:1004–1012. DOI: 10.1161/CIRCRESAHA.113.301198.

[34] O Joffre, MA Nolte, and R Spörri. Inflammatory signals in dendritic cell activation and the induction of adaptive immunity. Immunological Reviews. 2009; **227**:234–247. DOI: 10.1111/j.1600-065X.2008.00718.x.

[35] T Pentcheva-Hoang, JG Egen, K Wojnoonski, and JP Allison. B7-1 and B7-2 selectively recruit CTLA-4 and CD28 to the immunological synapse. Immunity. 2004; **21**:401–413. DOI: 10.1016/j.immuni.2004.06.017.

[36] A Ligers, N Teleshova, T Masterman, W Huang, and J Hillert. CTLA-4 gene expression is influenced by promoter and exon 1 polymorphisms. Genes and Immunity. 2001; **2**:145–152. DOI: 10.1038/sj.gene.6363752.

[37] EA Tivol, F Borriello, AN Schweitzer, WP Lynch, JA Bluestone, and AH Sharpe. Loss of CTLA-4 leads to massive lymphoproliferation and fatal multiorgan tissue destruction, revealing a critical negative regulatory role of CTLA-4. Immunity. 1995; **3**:541–547. DOI: 10.1016/1074-7613(95)90125-6.

[38] V Ruppert, T Meyer, C Struwe, J Petersen, A Perrot, MG Posch, C Özcelik, A Richter, B Maisch, and S Pankuweit. Evidence for CTLA4 as a susceptibility gene for dilated cardiomyopathy. European Journal of Human Genetics. 2010; **18**:694–699. DOI: 10.1038/ejhg.2010.3.

[39] T Kambayashi and TM Laufer. Atypical MHC class II-expressing antigen-presenting cells: can anything replace a dendritic cell? Nature Reviews Immunology. 2014; **14**:719–730. DOI: 10.1038/nri3754.

[40] AL Caforio, JT Stewart, E Bonifacio, M Burke, MJ Davies, WJ McKenna, and GF Bottazzo. Inappropriate major histocompatibility complex expression on cardiac tissue in dilated cardiomyopathy. Relevance for autoimmunity? Journal of Autoimmunity. 1990; **3**:187–200. DOI: 10.1016/0896-8411(90)90140-N.

[41] C Thelemann, S Haller, P Blyszczuk, G Kania, M Rosa, U Eriksson, S Rotman, W Reith, and H Acha-Orbea. Absence of nonhematopoietic MHC class II expression protects mice from experimental autoimmune myocarditis. European Journal of Immunology. 2015; **46**:656–664.

[42] AM Cordero-Reyes, KA Youker, AR Trevino, R Celis, DJ Hamilton, JH Flores-Arredondo, CM Orrego, A Bhimaraj, JD Estep, and G Torre-Amione. Full Expression of cardiomyopathy is partly dependent on B-cells: a pathway that involves cytokine activation, immunoglobulin deposition, and activation of apoptosis. Journal of the American Heart Association. 2016; **5**:e002484.

[43] H Nishimura, T Okazaki, Y Tanaka, K Nakatani, M Hara, A Matsumori, S Sasayama, A Mizoguchi, H Hiai, and N Minato. Autoimmune dilated cardiomyopathy in PD-1 receptor-deficient mice. Science. 2001; **291**:319–322. DOI: 10.1126/science.291.5502.319.

[44] M-L Thibult, E Mamessier, J Gertner-Dardenne, S Pastor, S Just-Landi, L Xerri, B Chetaille, and D Olive. PD-1 is a novel regulator of human B-cell activation. International Immunology. 2013; **25**:129–137. DOI: 10.1093/intimm/dxs098.

[45] KL Calame. Plasma cells: finding new light at the end of B cell development. Nature Immunology. 2001; **2**:1103–1108. DOI: 10.1038/ni1201-1103.

[46] J Yuan, M Yu, H-H Li, Q Long, W Liang, S Wen, M Wang, H-P Guo, X Cheng, and Y-H Liao. Autophagy contributes to IL-17-induced plasma cell differentiation in experimental autoimmune myocarditis. International Immunopharmacology. 2014; **18**:98–105. DOI: 10.1016/j.intimp.2013.11.008.

[47] AM Cordero-Reyes, KA Youker, and G Torre-Amione. The role of b-cells in heart failure. Methodist DeBakey Cardiovascular Journal. 2013; **9**:15–19. DOI: 10.14797/mdcj-9-1-15.

[48] R Jahns, V Boivin, L Hein, S Triebel, CE Angermann, G Ertl, and MJ Lohse. Direct evidence for a β 1-adrenergic receptor–directed autoimmune attack as a cause of idiopathic dilated cardiomyopathy. The Journal of Clinical Investigation. 2004; **113**:1419–1429. DOI: 10.1172/JCI20149.

[49] U Nussinovitch and Y Shoenfeld. The diagnostic and clinical significance of anti-muscarinic receptor autoantibodies. Clinical Reviews in Allergy & Immunology. 2012; **42**:298–308. DOI: 10.1007/s12016-010-8235-x.

[50] E Cunha-Neto, M Duranti, A Gruber, B Zingales, I De Messias, N Stolf, G Bellotti, ME Patarroyo, F Pilleggi, and J Kalil. Autoimmunity in Chagas disease cardiopathy: biological relevance of a cardiac myosin-specific epitope crossreactive to an immunodominant *Trypanosoma cruzi* antigen. Proceedings of the National Academy of Sciences. 1995; **92**:3541–3545.

[51] JC Silverio, LM De Oliveira Pinto, AA Da Silva, GM De Oliveira, and J Lannes-Vieira. Perforin-expressing cytotoxic cells contribute to chronic cardiomyopathy in *Trypanosoma cruzi* infection. International Journal of Experimental Pathology. 2010; **91**:72–86. DOI: 10.1111/j.1365-2613.2009.00670.x.

[52] JL Winters. Apheresis in the treatment of idiopathic dilated cardiomyopathy. Journal of Clinical Apheresis. 2012; **27**:312–319. DOI: 10.1002/jca.21245.

[53] A Baba and M Fu. Autoantibodies in atrial fibrillation: actor, biomarker or bystander? Autoimmunity. 2008; **41**:470–472. DOI: 10.1080/08916930802031504.

[54] SB Felix, A Staudt, M Landsberger, Y Grosse, V Stangl, T Spielhagen, G Wallukat, KD Wernecke, G Baumann, and K Stangl. Removal of cardiodepressant antibodies in dilated cardiomyopathy by immunoadsorption. Journal of the American College of Cardiology. 2002; **39**:646–652. DOI: 10.1016/S0735-1097(01)01794-6.

[55] J Chen, L Larsson, E Haugen, O Fedorkova, E Angwald, F Waagstein, and M Fu. Effects of autoantibodies removed by immunoadsorption from patients with dilated cardiomyopathy on neonatal rat cardiomyocytes. European Journal of Heart Failure. 2006; **8**:460–467. DOI: 10.1016/j.ejheart.2005.10.019.

[56] Y Staudt, C Trimpert, K Birkenmeier, T Krieg, T Bemmann, D Beug, S Felix, and A Staudt. Effects of antibodies obtained from patients with dilated cardiomyopathy on the function of isolated rat hearts. European Journal of Clinical Investigation. 2006; **36**:85–90. DOI: 10.1111/j.1365-2362.2006.01603.x.

[57] AL Caforio, A Angelini, M Blank, A Shani, S Kivity, G Goddard, A Doria, A Schiavo, M Testolina, and S Bottaro. Passive transfer of affinity-purified anti-heart autoantibodies (AHA) from sera of patients with myocarditis induces experimental myocarditis in mice. International Journal of Cardiology. 2015; **179**:166–177. DOI: 10.1016/j.ijcard.2014.10.165.

[58] CJ Limas, IF Goldenberg, and C Limas. Autoantibodies against beta-adrenoceptors in human idiopathic dilated cardiomyopathy. Circulation Research. 1989; **64**:97–103. DOI: 10.1161/01.RES.64.1.97.

[59] L-X Fu, Y Magnusson, C-H Bergh, J Liljeqvist, F Waagstein, A Hjalmarson, and J Hoebeke. Localization of a functional autoimmune epitope on the muscarinic acetylcholine receptor-2 in patients with idiopathic dilated cardiomyopathy. Journal of Clinical Investigation. 1993; **91**:1964–1968. DOI: 10.1172/JCI116416.

[60] R Klein, B Maisch, K Kochsiek, and P Berg. Demonstration of organ specific antibodies against heart mitochondria (anti-M7) in sera from patients with some forms of heart diseases. Clinical and Experimental Immunology. 1984; **58**:283–292.

[61] H-P Schultheiss. Dysfunction of the ADP/ATP carrier as a causative factor for the disturbance of the myocardial energy metabolism in dilated cardiomyopathy. Basic Research in Cardiology. 1992; **87**:311–320.

[62] N Neu, NR Rose, KW Beisel, A Herskowitz, G Gurri-Glass, and SW Craig. Cardiac myosin induces myocarditis in genetically predisposed mice. The Journal of Immunology. 1987; **139**:3630–3636.

[63] T Okazaki, Y Tanaka, R Nishio, T Mitsuiye, A Mizoguchi, J Wang, M Ishida, H Hiai, A Matsumori, and N Minato. Autoantibodies against cardiac troponin I are responsible

for dilated cardiomyopathy in PD-1-deficient mice. Nature Medicine. 2003; **9**:1477–1483. DOI: 10.1038/nm955.

[64] PG Wolff, U Kühl, and H-P Schultheiss. Laminin distribution and autoantibodies to laminin in dilated cardiomyopathy and myocarditis. American Heart Journal. 1989; **117**:1303–1309. DOI: 10.1016/0002-8703(89)90410-9.

[65] A-M Müller, M Bockstahler, G Hristov, C Weiß, A Fischer, S Korkmaz-Icöz, E Giannitsis, W Poller, H-P Schultheiss, and HA Katus. Identification of novel antigens contributing to autoimmunity in cardiovascular diseases. Clinical Immunology. 2016; **170**:30370–30379. DOI: 10.1016/j.clim.2016.09.003.

[66] A Baba, T Yoshikawa, and S Ogawa. Autoantibodies produced against sarcolemmal Na-K-ATPase: possible upstream targets of arrhythmias and sudden death in patients with dilated cardiomyopathy. Journal of the American College of Cardiology. 2002; **40**:1153–1159. DOI: 10.1016/S0735-1097(02)02075-2.

[67] N Latif, CS Baker, MJ Dunn, ML Rose, P Brady, and MH Yacoub. Frequency and specificity of antiheart antibodies in patients with dilated cardiomyopathy detected using SDS-PAGE and western blotting. Journal of the American College of Cardiology. 1993; **22**:1378–1384. DOI: 10.1016/0735-1097(93)90546-D.

[68] A Voigt, K Bartel, K Egerer, C Trimpert, E Feist, C Gericke, R Kandolf, K Klingel, U Kuckelkorn, and K Stangl. Humoral anti-proteasomal autoimmunity in dilated cardiomyopathy. Basic Research in Cardiology. 2010; **105**:9–18. DOI: 10.1007/s00395-009-0061-z.

[69] D Sánchez, P Gregor, K Čurila, I Hoffmanová, V Hábová, L Tučková, and H Tlaskalová-Hogenová. Anti-calreticulin antibodies and calreticulin in sera of patients diagnosed with dilated or hypertrophic cardiomyopathy. Autoimmunity. 2016; **30**:1–9. DOI: 10.1080/08916934.2016.1214822.

[70] Y Li, JS Heuser, LC Cunningham, SD Kosanke, and MW Cunningham. Mimicry and antibody-mediated cell signaling in autoimmune myocarditis. The Journal of Immunology. 2006; **177**:8234–8240. DOI: 10.4049/jimmunol.177.11.8234.

[71] M Afanasyeva, D Georgakopoulos, and NR Rose. Autoimmune myocarditis: cellular mediators of cardiac dysfunction. Autoimmunity Reviews. 2004; **3**:476–486. DOI: 10.1016/j.autrev.2004.08.009.

[72] U Eriksson, M Kurrer, R Bingisser, H Eugster, P Saremaslani, F Follath, S Marsch, and U Widmer. Lethal autoimmune myocarditis in interferon-γ receptor–deficient mice enhanced disease severity by impaired inducible nitric oxide synthase induction. Circulation. 2001; **103**:18–21. DOI: 10.1161/01.CIR.103.1.18.

[73] U Eriksson, MO Kurrer, N Schmitz, SC Marsch, A Fontana, H-P Eugster, and M Kopf. Interleukin-6–deficient mice resist development of autoimmune myocarditis associated with impaired upregulation of complement C3. Circulation. 2003; **107**:320–325. DOI: 10.1161/01.CIR.0000043802.38699.66.

[74] H Higuchi, M Hara, K Yamamoto, T Miyamoto, M Kinoshita, T Yamada, K Uchiyama, and A Matsumori. Mast cells play a critical role in the pathogenesis of viral myocarditis. Circulation. 2008; **118**:363–372. DOI: 10.1161/CIRCULATIONAHA.107.741595.

[75] T Nossuli, V Lakshminarayanan, G Baumgarten, G Taffet, C Ballantyne, L Michael, and M Entman. A chronic mouse model of myocardial ischemia-reperfusion: essential in cytokine studies. American Journal of Physiology-Heart and Circulatory Physiology. 2000; **278**:H1049–H1055.

[76] M Rangachari, N Mauermann, RR Marty, S Dirnhofer, MO Kurrer, V Komnenovic, JM Penninger, and U Eriksson. T-bet negatively regulates autoimmune myocarditis by suppressing local production of interleukin 17. The Journal of Experimental Medicine. 2006; **203**:2009–2019. DOI: 10.1084/jem.20052222.

[77] A Valaperti, RR Marty, G Kania, D Germano, N Mauermann, S Dirnhofer, B Leimenstoll, P Blyszczuk, C Dong, and C Mueller. CD11b+ monocytes abrogate Th17 CD4+ T cell-mediated experimental autoimmune myocarditis. The Journal of Immunology. 2008; **180**:2686–2695. DOI: 10.4049/jimmunol.180.4.2686.

[78] P Chen, G Baldeviano, D Ligons, M Talor, J Barin, N Rose, and D Cihakova. Susceptibility to autoimmune myocarditis is associated with intrinsic differences in CD4+ T cells. Clinical & Experimental Immunology. 2012; **169**:79–88. DOI: 10.1111/j.1365-2249.2012.04598.x.

[79] D Fairweather and D Cihakova. Alternatively activated macrophages in infection and autoimmunity. Journal of Autoimmunity. 2009; **33**:222–230. DOI: 10.1016/j.jaut.2009.09.012.

[80] N Rose. Critical cytokine pathways to cardiac inflammation. Journal of Interferon & Cytokine Research. 2011; **31**:705–710. DOI: 10.1089/jir.2011.0057.

[81] M Noutsias, M Rohde, K Göldner, A Block, K Blunert, L Hemaidan, M Hummel, JH Blohm, D Lassner, and U Kühl. Expression of functional T-cell markers and T-cell receptor Vbeta repertoire in endomyocardial biopsies from patients presenting with acute myocarditis and dilated cardiomyopathy. European Journal of Heart Failure. 2011; **13**:611–618.

[82] K Tajiri, N Shimojo, S Sakai, T Machino-Ohtsuka, K Imanaka-Yoshida, M Hiroe, Y Tsujimura, T Kimura, A Sato, and Y Yasutomi. Pitavastatin regulates helper T-cell differentiation and ameliorates autoimmune myocarditis in mice. Cardiovascular Drugs and Therapy. 2013; **27**:413–424. DOI: 10.1007/s10557-013-6464-y.

[83] SA Huber, AM Feldman, and D Sartini. Coxsackievirus B3 induces T regulatory cells, which inhibit cardiomyopathy in tumor necrosis factor-α transgenic mice. Circulation Research. 2006; **99**:1109–1116. DOI: 10.1161/01.RES.0000249405.13536.49.

[84] JT Chang, EJ Wherry, and AW Goldrath. Molecular regulation of effector and memory T cell differentiation. Nature Immunology. 2014; **15**:1104–1115. DOI: 10.1038/ni.3031.

[85] M Afanasyeva, Y Wang, Z Kaya, EA Stafford, KM Dohmen, AAS Akha, and NR Rose. Interleukin-12 receptor/STAT4 signaling is required for the development of

autoimmune myocarditis in mice by an interferon-γ-independent pathway. Circulation. 2001; **104**:3145–3151. DOI: 10.1161/hc5001.100629.

[86] GC Baldeviano, JG Barin, MV Talor, S Srinivasan, D Bedja, D Zheng, K Gabrielson, Y Iwakura, NR Rose, and D Cihakova. Interleukin-17A is dispensable for myocarditis but essential for the progression to dilated cardiomyopathy. Circulation Research. 2010; **106**:1646–1655. DOI: 10.1161/CIRCRESAHA.109.213157.

[87] V Nindl, R Maier, D Ratering, R De Giuli, R Züst, V Thiel, E Scandella, F Di Padova, M Kopf, and M Rudin. Cooperation of Th1 and Th17 cells determines transition from autoimmune myocarditis to dilated cardiomyopathy. European Journal of Immunology. 2012; **42**:2311–2321. DOI: 10.1002/eji.201142209.

[88] L Wu, NL Diny, S Ong, JG Barin, X Hou, NR Rose, MV Talor, and D Čiháková. Pathogenic IL-23 signaling is required to initiate GM-CSF-driven autoimmune myocarditis in mice. European journal of immunology. 2016; **46**:582–592.

[89] J Lane, DA Neumann, A Lafond-Walker, A Herskowitz, and NR Rose. Interleukin 1 or tumor necrosis factor can promote Coxsackie B3-induced myocarditis in resistant B10. A mice. The Journal of Experimental Medicine. 1992; **175**:1123–1129. DOI: 10.1084/jem.175.4.1123.

[90] D Neumann, J Lane, G Allen, A Herskowitz, and N Rose. Viral myocarditis leading to cardiomyopathy: do cytokines contribute to pathogenesis? Clinical Immunology and Immunopathology. 1993; **68**:181–190. DOI: 10.1006/clin.1993.1116.

[91] Y Wang, M Afanasyeva, SL Hill, Z Kaya, and NR Rose. Nasal administration of cardiac myosin suppresses autoimmune myocarditis in mice. Journal of the American College of Cardiology. 2000; **36**:1992–1999. DOI: 10.1016/S0735-1097(00)00939-6.

[92] A Awasthi and VK Kuchroo. Th17 cells: from precursors to players in inflammation and infection. International Immunology. 2009; **21**:489–498. DOI: 10.1093/intimm/dxp021.

[93] T Korn, E Bettelli, M Oukka, and VK Kuchroo. IL-17 and Th17 Cells. Annual Review of Immunology. 2009; **27**:485–517. DOI: 10.1146/annurev.immunol.021908.132710.

[94] JM Myers, LT Cooper, DC Kem, S Stavrakis, SD Kosanke, EM Shevach, D Fairweather, JA Stoner, CJ Cox, and MW Cunningham. Cardiac myosin-Th17 responses promote heart failure in human myocarditis. JCI Insight. 2016; **1**.

[95] Y Lee, A Awasthi, N Yosef, FJ Quintana, S Xiao, A Peters, C Wu, M Kleinewietfeld, S Kunder, and DA Hafler. Induction and molecular signature of pathogenic Th17 cells. Nature Immunology. 2012; **13**:991–999. DOI: 10.1038/ni.2416.

[96] A Beringer, M Noack, and P Miossec. IL-17 in chronic inflammation: from discovery to targeting. Trends in Molecular Medicine. 2016; **22**:230–241. DOI: 10.1016/j.molmed.2016.01.001.

[97] S Rutz, C Eidenschenk, JR Kiefer, and W Ouyang. Post-translational regulation of RORγt—A therapeutic target for the modulation of interleukin-17-mediated responses

in autoimmune diseases. Cytokine & Growth Factor Reviews. 2016; **30**:1–17. DOI: 10.1016/j.cytogfr.2016.07.004.

[98] ML Diller, RR Kudchadkar, KA Delman, DH Lawson, and ML Ford. Balancing inflammation: The link between Th17 and regulatory T cells. Mediators of Inflammation. 2016; **2016**: 6309219-6309227. DOI:10.1155/2016/6309219..

[99] L Zhon, J Lopes, and M Chong. TGF-beta-induced Foxp3 inhibits Thl7 cell differentiation by antagonizing ROR gamma function E J. Nature. 2008; **453**:236–240.

[100] N Komatsu, K Okamoto, S Sawa, T Nakashima, M Oh-Hora, T Kodama, S Tanaka, JA Bluestone, and H Takayanagi. Pathogenic conversion of Foxp3+ T cells into Th17 cells in autoimmune arthritis. Nature Medicine. 2014; **20**:62–68. DOI: 10.1038/nm.3432.

[101] S Okada, H Inoue, K Yamauchi, H Iijima, Y Ohkawara, T Takishima, and K Shirato. Potential role of interleukin-1 in allergen-induced late asthmatic reactions in guinea pigs: suppressive effect of interleukin-1 receptor antagonist on late asthmatic reaction. Journal of Allergy and Clinical Immunology. 1995; **95**:1236–1245. DOI: 10.1016/S0091-6749(95)70081-1.

[102] PK Dagur, A Biancotto, E Stansky, HN Sen, RB Nussenblatt, and JP McCoy. Secretion of interleukin-17 by CD8+ T cells expressing CD146 (MCAM). Clinical Immunology. 2014; **152**:36–47. DOI: 10.1016/j.clim.2014.01.009.

[103] U Srenathan, K Steel, and LS Taams. IL-17+ CD8+ T cells: Differentiation, phenotype and role in inflammatory disease. Immunology Letters. 2016.

[104] A Xin, F Masson, Y Liao, S Preston, T Guan, R Gloury, M Olshansky, J-X Lin, P Li, and TP Speed. A molecular threshold for effector CD8+ T cell differentiation controlled by transcription factors Blimp-1 and T-bet. Nature Immunology. 2016. DOI: 10.1038/ni.3410.

[105] JC Gasson. Molecular physiology of granulocyte-macrophage colony-stimulating factor. Blood. 1991; **77**:1131–1145.

[106] I Sonderegger, G Iezzi, R Maier, N Schmitz, M Kurrer, and M Kopf. GM-CSF mediates autoimmunity by enhancing IL-6–dependent Th17 cell development and survival. The Journal of Experimental Medicine. 2008; **205**:2281–2294. DOI: 10.1084/jem.20071119.

[107] H Chang, H Hanawa, T Yoshida, M Hayashi, H Liu, L Ding, K Otaki, K Hao, K Yoshida, and K Kato. Alteration of IL-17 related protein expressions in experimental autoimmune myocarditis and inhibition of IL-17 by IL-10-Ig fusion gene transfer. Circulation Journal. 2008; **72**:813–819. DOI: 10.1253/circj.72.813.

[108] DM Cortez, MD Feldman, S Mummidi, AJ Valente, B Steffensen, M Vincenti, JL Barnes, and B Chandrasekar. IL-17 stimulates MMP-1 expression in primary human cardiac fibroblasts via p38 MAPK-and ERK1/2-dependent C/EBP-β, NF-κB, and AP-1 activation. American Journal of Physiology-Heart and Circulatory Physiology. 2007; **293**:H3356–H3365. DOI: 10.1152/ajpheart.00928.2007.

[109] A Doreau, A Belot, J Bastid, B Riche, M-C Trescol-Biemont, B Ranchin, N Fabien, P Cochat, C Pouteil-Noble, and P Trolliet. Interleukin 17 acts in synergy with B cell–activating factor to influence B cell biology and the pathophysiology of systemic lupus erythematosus. Nature Immunology. 2009; **10**:778–785. DOI: 10.1038/ni.1741.

[110] I Sonderegger, TA Röhn, MO Kurrer, G Iezzi, Y Zou, RA Kastelein, MF Bachmann, and M Kopf. Neutralization of IL-17 by active vaccination inhibits IL-23-dependent autoimmune myocarditis. European Journal of Immunology. 2006; **36**:2849–2856.

[111] T Yamashita, T Iwakura, K Matsui, H Kawaguchi, M Obana, A Hayama, M Maeda, Y Izumi, I Komuro, and Y Ohsugi. IL-6-mediated Th17 differentiation through RORγt is essential for the initiation of experimental autoimmune myocarditis. Cardiovascular Research. 2011; **91**:640–648. DOI: 10.1093/cvr/cvr148.

[112] J Yuan, A-L Cao, M Yu, Q-W Lin, X Yu, J-H Zhang, M Wang, H-P Guo, and Y-H Liao. Th17 cells facilitate the humoral immune response in patients with acute viral myocarditis. Journal of Clinical Immunology. 2010; **30**:226–234. DOI: 10.1007/s10875-009-9355-z.

[113] PM da Matta Guedes, FR Gutierrez, FL Maia, CM Milanezi, GK Silva, WR Pavanelli, and JS Silva. IL-17 produced during *Trypanosoma cruzi* infection plays a central role in regulating parasite-induced myocarditis. PLoS Neglected Tropical Disease. 2010; **4**:e604. DOI: 10.1371/journal.pntd.0000604.

[114] JT Boari, MCA Vesely, DA Bermejo, MC Ramello, CL Montes, H Cejas, A Gruppi, and EVA Rodríguez. IL-17RA signaling reduces inflammation and mortality during *Trypanosoma cruzi* infection by recruiting suppressive IL-10-producing neutrophils. PLoS Pathogens 2012; **8**:e1002658.

[115] PM Da Matta Guedes, FRS Gutierrez, GK Silva, R Dellalibera-Joviliano, GJ Rodrigues, LM Bendhack, A Rassi Jr, A Rassi, A Schmidt, and BC Maciel. Deficient regulatory T cell activity and low frequency of IL-17-producing T cells correlate with the extent of cardiomyopathy in human Chagas' disease. PLoS Neglected Tropical Disease. 2012; **6**:e1630. DOI: 10.1371/journal.pntd.0001630.

[116] T Simon, S Taleb, N Danchin, L Laurans, B Rousseau, S Cattan, J-M Montely, O Dubourg, A Tedgui, and S Kotti. Circulating levels of interleukin-17 and cardiovascular outcomes in patients with acute myocardial infarction. European Heart Journal. 2012; **34**:570–577. DOI: 10.1093/eurheartj/ehs263.

[117] CG Martinez, D Zamith-Miranda, MG da Silva, KC Ribeiro, IT Brandão, CL Silva, BL Diaz, M Bellio, PM Persechini, and E Kurtenbach. P2× 7 purinergic signaling in dilated cardiomyopathy induced by auto-immunity against muscarinic M2 receptors: autoantibody levels, heart functionality and cytokine expression. Scientific reports. 2015; **5**.

[118] JR Schoenborn and CB Wilson. Regulation of interferon-γ during innate and adaptive immune responses. Advances in immunology. 2007; **96**:41–101.

[119] O Meyer. Interferons and autoimmune disorders. Joint Bone Spine. 2009; **76**:464–473. DOI: 10.1016/j.jbspin.2009.03.012.

[120] PS de Araújo-Souza, SC Hanschke, and JP Viola. Epigenetic control of interferon-gamma expression in CD8 T cells. Journal of Immunology Research. 2015; **2015**:1–7. DOI: 10.1155/2015/849573.

[121] SJ Szabo, BM Sullivan, SL Peng, and LH Glimcher. Molecular mechanisms regulating Th1 immune responses. Annual Review of Immunology. 2003; **21**:713–758. DOI: 10.1146/annurev.immunol.21.120601.140942.

[122] LK Teixeira, BP Fonseca, A Vieira-de-Abreu, BA Barboza, BK Robbs, PT Bozza, and JP Viola. IFN-γ production by CD8+ T cells depends on NFAT1 transcription factor and regulates Th differentiation. The Journal of Immunology. 2005; **175**:5931–5939. DOI: 10.4049/jimmunol.175.9.5931.

[123] L Baudino, SA da Silveira, M Nakata, and S Izui. Molecular and cellular basis for pathogenicity of autoantibodies: lessons from murine monoclonal autoantibodies. Springer Seminars in Immunopathology. 2006; **28**:175–184. DOI: 10.1007/s00281-006-0037-0.

[124] X Hu and LB Ivashkiv. Cross-regulation of signaling pathways by interferon-γ: implications for immune responses and autoimmune diseases. Immunity. 2009; **31**:539–550. DOI: 10.1016/j.immuni.2009.09.002.

[125] D Bending, H De La Peña, M Veldhoen, JM Phillips, C Uyttenhove, B Stockinger, and A Cooke. Highly purified Th17 cells from BDC2. 5NOD mice convert into Th1-like cells in NOD/SCID recipient mice. The Journal of Clinical Investigation. 2009; **119**:565–572. DOI: 10.1172/JCI37865.

[126] K Boniface, WM Blumenschein, K Brovont-Porth, MJ McGeachy, B Basham, B Desai, R Pierce, TK McClanahan, S Sadekova, and R de Waal Malefyt. Human Th17 cells comprise heterogeneous subsets including IFN-γ-producing cells with distinct properties from the Th1 lineage. The Journal of Immunology. 2010; **185**:679–687. DOI: 10.4049/jimmunol.1000366.

[127] R Baccala, DH Kono, and AN Theofilopoulos. Interferons as pathogenic effectors in autoimmunity. Immunological Reviews. 2005; **204**:9–26. DOI: 10.1111/j.0105-2896.2005.00252.x.

[128] SP Levick and PH Goldspink. Could interferon-gamma be a therapeutic target for treating heart failure? Heart Failure Reviews. 2014; **19**:227–236. DOI: 10.1007/s10741-013-9393-8.

[129] M Afanasyeva, D Georgakopoulos, DF Belardi, D Bedja, D Fairweather, Y Wang, Z Kaya, KL Gabrielson, ER Rodriguez, and P Caturegli. Impaired up-regulation of CD25 on CD4+ T cells in IFN-γ knockout mice is associated with progression of myocarditis to heart failure. Proceedings of the National Academy of Sciences of the United States of America. 2005; **102**:180–185. DOI: 10.1073/pnas.0408241102.

[130] M Afanasyeva, Y Wang, Z Kaya, S Park, MJ Zilliox, BH Schofield, SL Hill, and NR Rose. Experimental autoimmune myocarditis in A/J mice is an interleukin-4-dependent disease with a Th2 phenotype. The American Journal of Pathology. 2001; **159**:193–203. DOI: 10.1016/S0002-9440(10)61685-9.

[131] JG Barin, GC Baldeviano, MV Talor, L Wu, S Ong, D Fairweather, D Bedja, NR Stickel, JA Fontes, and AB Cardamone. Fatal Eosinophilic Myocarditis Develops in the Absence of IFN-γ and IL-17A. The Journal of Immunology. 2013; **191**:4038–4047. DOI: 10.4049/jimmunol.1301282.

[132] G Kania, S Siegert, S Behnke, R Prados-Rosales, A Casadevall, TF Lüscher, SA Luther, M Kopf, U Eriksson, and P Blyszczuk. Innate signaling promotes formation of regulatory nitric oxide-producing dendritic cells limiting T-cell expansion in experimental autoimmune myocarditis. Circulation. 2013; **127**:2285–2294. DOI: 10.1161/CIRCULATIONAHA.112.000434.

[133] A Furrer, MO Hottiger, and A Valaperti. Absent in melanoma 2 (AIM2) limits proinflammatory cytokine transcription in cardiomyocytes by inhibiting STAT1 phosphorylation. Molecular Immunology. 2016; **74**:47–58. DOI: 10.1016/j.molimm.2016.04.009.

[134] CM Cascabulho, DG Beghini, M Meuser-Batista, C Penido, and A Henriques-Pons. Chemotaxis and immunoregulatory function of cardiac $\gamma\delta$ T cells in dystrophin-deficient mice. The Journal of Immunology. 2016:1600335. DOI: 10.4049/jimmunol.1600335.

[135] C Massilamany, A Gangaplara, RH Basavalingappa, RA Rajasekaran, V Khalilzad-Sharghi, Z Han, S Othman, D Steffen, and J Reddy. Localization of CD8 T cell epitope within cardiac myosin heavy chain-α 334–352 that induces autoimmune myocarditis in A/J mice. International Journal of Cardiology. 2016; **202**:311–321. DOI: 10.1016/j.ijcard.2015.09.016.

[136] P Blyszczuk, C Berthonneche, S Behnke, M Glönkler, H Moch, T Pedrazzini, TF Lüscher, U Eriksson, and G Kania. Nitric oxide synthase 2 is required for conversion of profibrogenic inflammatory CD133+ progenitors into F4/80+ macrophages in experimental autoimmune myocarditis. Cardiovascular Research. 2013; **97**:219–229. DOI: 10.1093/cvr/cvs317.

[137] S Ong, DL Ligons, JG Barin, L Wu, MV Talor, N Diny, JA Fontes, E Gebremariam, DA Kass, and NR Rose. Natural killer cells limit cardiac inflammation and fibrosis by halting eosinophil infiltration. The American Journal of Pathology. 2015; **185**:847–861. DOI: 10.1016/j.ajpath.2014.11.023.

[138] NL Diny, X Hou, JG Barin, G Chen, MV Talor, J Schaub, SD Russell, K Klingel, NR Rose, and D Čiháková. Macrophages and cardiac fibroblasts are the main producers of eotaxins and regulate eosinophil trafficking to the heart. European Journal of Immunology. 2016. DOI: 10.1002/eji.201646557.

[139] T Weinberger and C Schulz. Myocardial infarction: a critical role of macrophages in cardiac remodeling. Frontiers in Physiology. 2015; **6**:107. DOI: 10.3389/fphys.2015.00107.

[140] M Nahrendorf and FK Swirski. Monocyte and macrophage heterogeneity in the heart. Circulation Research. 2013; **112**:1624–1633. DOI: 10.1161/CIRCRESAHA.113.300890.

[141] G De Couto, W Liu, E Tseliou, B Sun, N Makkar, H Kanazawa, M Arditi, and E Marbán. Macrophages mediate cardioprotective cellular postconditioning in acute myocardial

infarction. The Journal of Clinical Investigation. 2015; **125**:3147–3162. DOI: 10.1172/JCI81321.

[142] O Zimmermann, JM Homann, A Bangert, A-M Müller, G Hristov, S Goeser, JM Wiehe, S Zittrich, W Rottbauer, and J Torzewski. Successful use of mRNA-nucleofection for overexpression of interleukin-10 in murine monocytes/macrophages for anti-inflammatory therapy in a murine model of autoimmune myocarditis. Journal of the American Heart Association. 2012; **1**:e003293. DOI: 10.1161/JAHA.112.003293.

[143] D Cihakova, JG Barin, M Afanasyeva, M Kimura, D Fairweather, M Berg, MV Talor, GC Baldeviano, S Frisancho, and K Gabrielson. Interleukin-13 protects against experimental autoimmune myocarditis by regulating macrophage differentiation. The American Journal of Pathology. 2008; **172**:1195–1208. DOI: 10.2353/ajpath.2008.070207.

[144] S Gao, J Zhou, N Liu, L Wang, Q Gao, Y Wu, Q Zhao, P Liu, S Wang, and Y Liu. Curcumin induces M2 macrophage polarization by secretion IL-4 and/or IL-13. Journal of Molecular and Cellular Cardiology. 2015; **85**:131–139. DOI: 10.1016/j.yjmcc.2015.04.025.

[145] Z Su, P Zhang, Y Yu, H Lu, Y Liu, P Ni, X Su, D Wang, Y Liu, and J Wang. HMGB1 Facilitated macrophage reprogramming towards a proinflammatory M1-like phenotype in experimental autoimmune myocarditis development. Scientific Reports. 2016; **6**. DOI: 10.1038/srep21884.

Chapter 5

Autoimmunity of Gastrointestinal Tract

Anna Pituch-Noworolska and
Monika Mach-Tomalska

Additional information is available at the end of the chapter

http://dx.doi.org/10.5772/67281

Abstract

Gastrointestinal tract diseases are recognised as autoimmune based on typical histopathology, presence of autoantibodies in serum and clinical response to immunosuppressive therapy. Like in other autoimmune diseases, the inducing factor is unknown; however, accumulating data suggests an increasing role of microbiota homeostasis and relation between the immune system (mucous-associated lymphoid tissue) and microbiota in intestinal lumen. The inflammation process is now described as autoinflammation with inflammasome formation or autoimmune chronic inflammation with overproduction of pro-inflammatory cytokines. Diagnostic procedures include autoantibodies assay, histology of biopsy from intestinal mucous, genetic background (especially in celiac disease) and clinical symptoms. Therapy is adjusted to pathomechanism including regulation of microbiota homeostasis with pre-biotics and probiotics, inhibition of inflammatory process with steroids, classical immunosuppression and anti-cytokine monoclonal antibodies and haematopoietic stem cells transplantation in severe cases with therapy resistance, progression and life-threatening course. The aim of this chapter is to review mechanisms of autoinflammation and autoimmunity, diagnosis and therapy of gastrointestinal tract.

Keywords: autoimmunity, autoinflammation, microbiota homeostasis, pro-inflammatory cytokines, autoantibodies, immunosuppression, monoclonal antibodies

1. Introduction

Autoimmunity is the aberrant reaction of specific immune system to autoantigens. The stimuli leading to recognition of own determinants, receptors, cell products as antigens, followed by activation of T and B lymphocytes are unknown. The genetic background is described in few diseases from a long list of autoimmune syndromes. This aberrant reaction of immune system is irreversible, so the diagnosis of autoimmune process makes it lifelong one. The criteria of autoimmune process include tissue infiltration with immunocompetent cells, overproduction of pro-inflammatory cytokines, and production of autoantibodies by plasmocytes. This process is going for years before clinical manifestation as an effect of non-reparable tissue damage. Autoimmune diseases are classified as systemic or organ-specific, based on origin of autoantigen and involved organs being the target for autoantibodies and deposits of immune complexes binding and activating complement cascade. The presence of autoantibodies in serum is one of the laboratory criteria for the ongoing autoimmune process; moreover, the precise description of the type and amount of autoantibodies suggests the type of disease. The aim of this chapter is to review mechanisms of autoinflammation and autoimmunity, diagnosis and therapy of gastrointestinal tract.

2. Physiology of gastrointestinal tract mucous membrane

2.1. The role of microbiota

In our intestinal lumen exists about 10^{14} commensal organisms is in symbiotic relation with the host. The interaction of microbiota and intestinal immune system including innate and adoptive immune mechanisms is bidirectional—microorganisms are influencing activity of cells present in epithelial cell monolayer and activity of immune cells is regulating commensal microbiota compound, localization and attachment to epithelial cells [1, 2]. The newborn babies acquire the microbiota during vaginal birth. It is obvious that caesarean section obviates contact with vaginal microenvironment and that resulted in differences of microbiota. The colonization of intestine at birth affects innate and adaptive immune system associated with mucous membrane of gut [3]. The response of immune system differentiating between commensal and invasive pathogens is not fully elucidated yet. The role of toll-like receptors (TLR), especially TLR5 for bacterial flagellin, is described based on inflammation in deficiency of this receptor. TRLs are pathogen recognition sensors detecting bacterias, viruses and fungi. Stimulation of TLRs and NOD-like receptors (NLRs) leads to the production of pro-inflammatory cytokines and formation of protein complex called inflammasome. NLRs are the group of intra-cellular pattern recognitions receptors (PRRs) involved in the recognition of many DAMPs and PAPMs (danger and pathogen-associated molecular patterns) in commensal and pathogenic microbiota. Inflammasome is a crucial structure for defence to pathogens but, from the other perspective, is involved in pathogenesis of autoinflammatory and autoimmune diseases following the prolonged inflammatory process [4–6]. The forming of inflammasome is not the only way of interaction between microbiota and immune systems. Another is based on influence of bacterial metabolites and its components such as fatty acids on epithelial cells inducing production of antimicrobial peptides (AMP). Stimulated epithelial cells produce IL-25 directly reacting with myeloid cells present in mucous. The cascade of activation resulted in stimulation of ILC3 subpopulation of immune system and production of cytokines [5].

2.2. The immune system of mucous membrane

The mucous membrane is one of our defence mechanisms against pathogenic microorganism intake with food into intestinal lumen. Its basic role is to regulate the response of immune

http://dx.doi.org/10.5772/67281

system to pathogens and the homeostasis of commensal microbiota. The epithelial layer consists of different cells like epithelial cells, M cells, Paneth cells and goblet cells with specific function of mucous production. There are differences of stages of *in situ* maturating along transposition from crypts to the surface of epithelial layer. Moreover, some observations suggest the cross-talk between epithelial cells and commensal microbiota facilitating to maintain homeostasis and to improve response to infectious pathogens. Paneth cells are localized close to crypts in the villi of small intestine. The expression of MyD88 molecule is important for TLR-MyD88-dependent pathway of microbiota recognition. Stimulation of this way results in the production of antimicrobial factors such as defensin, CRP-ductin, RegIII-γ and others to protect the optimal environment for crypts' stem cells. The goblet cells are also regulated partially through TLRs. The main role of goblet cells is production of mucins inhibiting the attachment of bacterial (commensal or pathogenic) to epithelial cells layer, particularly mucin-2, a main colonic gel-forming one [5]. The role of M cells is based on uptake of antigens from luminal spaces and induction of antigen-specific immune response. Their localization in the follicles-associated epithelia of Payer's patches and/or isolated lymphoid follicles facilitates the induction of antigen-specific immune response within the mucous membrane. The last study showed that M cells are the entry point for intra-tissues commensal flora inducing IgA production in Peyer's patches [5, 7]. The last equally important cells from epithelial layer are columnar epithelial cells forming very tight monolayer surface barrier, being regulated by the commensal microbiota. The role of bridge between the innate and adaptive immune systems in mucous membrane plays interleukin 23 (IL-23). The axis IL-23/IL-17 is important for IL-17 producing cells-Th17 subpopulation of T lymphocytes. In mucosal sites, the cell populations consist of T lymphocytes derived mainly from TCRγ/δ subpopulation, Th17 lymphocytes, mature T lymphocytes TCRα/β (CD3/CD4, CD3/CD8) and dendritic cells, NK cells. IL-23 induces cytokines production by innate lymphoid cells (ILCs) discovered in the mucous system. ILCs belong to three different types—group 1: ILC1 and NK cells producing IFN-γ, group 2: ILC2 natural helper cells expressing retinoid acid receptor (RAR) and group 3: ILC3 including foetal lymphoid tissue inducer cells, subpopulation of NK cells (NK22, NKp46 positive/negative). ILCs produce IL-17A, IL-17F or IL-22. These groups differ in expression of receptors and, in consequence, play different regulatory roles in maintaining the homeostasis, induction of immune system response and inflammatory process [4, 5]. Th17 lymphocytes, localized in lamina propria, produce large amounts of cytokines: IL-17A, IL-17F, IL-21 and IL-22 after stimulation with IL-6 and TGF-β. Increased expression of IL-23 receptor on Th17 lymphocytes induces positive autoregulatory feedback loop. Cytokines produced by Th17 clear microbes reaching lamina propria, maintain tightness of mucous barrier [2]. This subpopulation of T lymphocytes is very important in induction of inflammation, so the regulation of functions inhibits or induces this process. Moreover, within T lymphocytes was described small subpopulation with phenotype CD3/CD4/CD25 and FoxP3 called T regulatory cell with main function of regulation and control of the autoimmune process. Those Tregs are main producers of anti-inflammatory cytokines—IL-10 and TGF-β balancing pro-inflammatory derived activation of cells [2, 4, 5, 7]. The low number or dysfunction of these cells facilitates autoimmunity development. Those, depletion of Treg may explain the high frequency of autoimmune diseases among patients with humoral immunity deficiencies.

2.3. The role of IgA

Dimeric, secretory IgA (sIgA) is produced locally by B cells and plasma cells present in lamina propria, isolated lymphoid follicles (ILF) and subepithelial dome (SED) of Peyer's patches in intestine wall. The J chain (joining chain) responsible for the dimeric structure of IgA contributes in binding of IgA to polymeric immunoglobulin receptor (pIgR) facilitating the transport through epithelial cells and release into intestinal lumen. The data about the role of sIgA systematically increase based on clinical symptoms and disturbances of gut microbiota homeostasis in patients with isolated IgA deficiency when IgG and IgM are replacing sIgA. Now, the sIgA role is well known. Molecules of sIgA bind to pathogens and block the attachment to epithelial cells and invasion into intestinal tissue. This activity of sIgA, called immunological exclusion, is very effective in defence of epithelial cells during the mucosal infections [8]. Moreover, IgA facilitates contact of the different particles from intestinal lumen with dendritic cells localized in SED of Peyer's patches. IgA also plays a regulating role for commensal microbiota with large fraction coated with IgA in normal, homeostatic conditions [8]. Plasmablast-producing IgA is generated locally in GALT from naïve B cell, mainly in Peyer's patches. IgA plasmablast migrates into intestinal lamina propria and maturates into IgA-antibody secreting cells (IgA-ASC) along this way. The regulation of this migration is based on the combination of cytokines and adhesion molecules expression e.g. CCR9 and CCR10—mucosa-specific chemokine receptors on IgA-ASC. The expression of ligands for these receptors showed different patterns depending on localization in intestine—jejunum or large bowel. Moreover, the types of antigens and their stimulation of IgA production are important for regulating IgA-dependent response in different parts of intestine. IgA production and maturation of plasmablasts are regulated by T cell–derived cytokines. T lymphocytes are involved in the formation of germinal centres and generation of IgA producing cells through, e.g., induction of activation-induced cytidine deaminase (AID) expression in B lymphocytes. This enzyme is critical for the process of a class switch recombination and hypermutation leading to production of IgA. Subpopulations of T cells—Th17 and Treg cells—play the special regulatory role for IgA transport through induction of expression of polymeric immunoglobulin (pIgR) receptor on epithelial cells. In promotion of IgA-producing cells, the following cytokines T lymphocytes-derived are involved—TGF-β, IL-4, IL-10 and IL-21. TGF-β acts on B lymphocytes as a promoter of naïve B cell proliferation and maturation, where IL-21 promotes the generation of IgA plasmablasts. The best effect on IgA production is noted when both cytokines are present and acts synergistically [9, 10].

3. Mechanisms of autoinflammatory process

3.1. The inflammation as a process occurs at the following situations

- First—acute response of immune system to pathogens invading the tissue after breaking the natural defence e.g. epithelial cells layer of mucous membrane etc. This process is terminated after elimination of pathogens with subsequent healing of damaged tissue process.

- Second—prolonged response due to recurrent fever episodes, recurrent inflammasome formation and overproduction of pro-inflammatory cytokines mediated by innate immune system. Here it belongs to a wide range of periodic fever syndromes. Nowadays, it is suggested, that Crohn's disease, as the result of aberrant bacterial sensing, is fulfilling the criteria of autoinflammatory process.

- Third—chronic inflammatory reactions with production of autoantibodies against tissue and/or cellular elements resulting with irreversible damage of cells, tissues and organs. This self-directed and sustained chronic inflammation is typical for autoimmunity, mediated by adaptive immune system, immune complexes formation and complement activation [6, 11–13].

3.2. Inflammasome and innate immune system

The receptors of innate immunity components (cells) reacting with pathogen molecular patterns are called—pathogen patterns recognition receptors (PRRs). PRRs are reacting with pathogen-associated molecular patterns (PAMPs) and danger-associated molecular patterns (DAMPs). Within different types of PRRs, most important for inflammasome formation are ones from the nucleotide-binding domain leucine-rich repeat (NLRs) family. In human this family contains 22 genes, but the formation of inflammasomes (large protein complex) is associated with NLRP3, NLRP1, NLRC4 and AIM2. Inflammasome is a mediator of autoactivation of Caspase-1 and that in turn leads to activation of IL-1b and IL-18 [6, 13]. The inflammatory process with the inflammasome formation is associated with activation of neutrophils, monocytes and macrophages. Among the chronic inflammatory diseases of the gastrointestinal tract, Crohn's disease seems to be mediated by autoinflammatory than autoimmune pathomechanisms.

3.3. From autoinflammation to autoimmunity

The products of inflammasome such as IL-1β and IL-18 influence not only innate immune system but also adaptive system, through activation of T and B lymphocytes. The up-regulation of IL-2 R (receptor for IL-2) expression on T cells, boosts of B cells–derived production of antibodies, supports prolonged survival of T and B lymphocytes. The other effects of these cytokines is acceleration of Th17 (by IL-1β) and Th1 (by IL-18), functional subpopulations of T cells, maturation [6]. The activity of overproduced cytokines in inflammasome bridges the innate and adaptive immunity system in reactions to pathogens. Apparently, there are some diseases with pathomechanisms of both types of chronic inflammatory reactions as a continuum from typical autoinflammatory to autoimmune disease. This hypothesis formed by Kastner [12] was based on shift of components of tissue infiltrations along the time of disease—during autoinflammatory stages, the majority of cells were—neutrophils, monocytes, macrophages and dendritic cells—smoothly transforming to infiltration typical for autoimmune process such as activated T and B lymphocytes producing typical profiles of cytokines, e.g. Th1, Th17 and autoantibodies [12].

4. Mechanisms of autoimmunity

4.1. Activity of immunocompetent cells and overproduction of cytokines

Mechanisms of supporting the self-tolerance are based on suppression of effector T lymphocytes proliferation and down-regulation of immune response [14]. The peripheral tolerance is regulated with different mechanisms, but a crucial role in maintaining this tolerance is played by regulatory T cells (Tregs). The dysfunction and/or decreased number of Tregs is associated with increased risk of autoimmunity, seen as a case in patients with humoral immunodeficiency (e.g. CVID), where more than 60% of patients demonstrate a low number of Tregs and co-existent autoimmune diseases such as diabetes mellitus type 1, systemic lupus erythematousus, celiac disease, thyroid diseases, etc. Naive Tregs are generated in thymus and transformed to inducible Treg (iTreg) in periphery, mainly in the gut. Tregs produce anti-inflammatory cytokines—TGF-β1, IL-10, IL-35 [14–16]. Immune response to pathogens includes differentiation of T lymphocytes into two functional subpopulations—T helper 1 (Th1) producing pro-inflammatory cytokines and T helper 2 (Th2) producing anti-inflammatory cytokines. Additional subpopulations of T lymphocytes are Th17 cells releasing IL-17 (IL-17A, IL-17F). The list of cytokines derived from cells involved in pathogens' response is long, and among them, cytokines such as TNF and IL-22 also play an important role.

Activation of Th1 lymphocytes results in high level of IFN-γ and IL-2 and/or TNF. The Th1-derived profile of cytokines supports inflammation and induces fever and infiltrations in target tissues. Intra-cellular bacterias and micobacterias are killed by macrophages activated with Th17-derived cytokines [16, 17]. Th2 subpopulation balances pro-inflammatory cytokines activity due to anti-inflammatory suppressing role of IL-4, IL-5 and IL-13 [14–16]. The profile of cytokines typical for given subpopulation of Th cells is not limited and Th2 are producing small amount of TNF and IL-2 with pro-inflammatory activity. Stimulation of B cells towards immunoglobulins class switching is also associated with Th2 cells [16]. Stimulated B lymphocytes produce specific antibodies either, differentiate into memory cells subpopulation or mature into plasmablast and long-life plasmocytes. In terms of autoimmunity B cell differentiation and maturation is directed to autoantigens and result in autoantibodies production.

In last few years dysfunction of autophagy was declared a new crucial mechanism for development of inflammatory bowel diseases. In physiology autophagy is one of cellular stress response indispensable for adaptation to starvation, degradation of aberrant proteins or organelles. Moreover, genes loci associated with increased risk for IBD are shared with genes required for autophagy, suggesting possibility of autophagy disorders in IBD. In mucous membrane function, the disorders of autophagy affect some aspects of innate and acquired inflammatory response, e.g. function of Paneth cells, cytokines production, pathogens clearance and, what was showed in last time, decrease function of goblet cells and absorptive function of microvilli [18, 19].

4.2. Production and role of autoantibodies

The natural antibodies of IgM class with moderate self-antigen affinity play first-line role in defence against pathogens. The autoantibodies showing high affinity to our own antigens are

IgG class and are concerned as pathologic, although they are detected in low titres in serum of healthy individuals [20]. The reaction of IgG autoantibodies with antigens, circulating in serum or present in tissue, forms complexes activating complement pathway. Complement activation mediating tissue damage is concerned in systemic autoimmune disease e.g. SLE, less expressed in organ-specific diseases, when antibodies react with target antigen presented in given organ e.g. thyroid, Langerhans islet or suprarenal gland cells, ovary cells and others. Beside the role in tissue damage process, the presence of autoantibodies is the marker of autoimmune process and/or mechanism leading to clinical symptoms. Type and titre of antibodies circulating in serum support clinical diagnosis and help in differential diagnosis of overlapping syndromes. Association of autoantibody levels with clinical course of disease is rare, but important for therapy adjustment e.g. dsDNA level in SLE. In systemic autoimmune diseases the role of B-1 subset of B lymphocytes in autoantibodies production was suggested due to high effectiveness of B-1 cells in presenting antigen process [20]. The long list of different types of autoantibodies reflects the long list of structures inducing antigen-dependent B cells response. Autoantibodies against nuclear proteins and organelles are believed to be a consequence of exposing previously hidden antigens due to apoptosis, the presence of cell debris and disturbances of dying cell cleavage. The good example for cell debris serving as antigen is production of antibodies to cyclic citrullinated peptides (CCP) in rheumatoid arthritis as a result of acquired neoepitope after prolonged inflammation. The autoantibodies used as a marker of autoimmune disease are helpful in diagnosis in overt disease; however, they are present also in detectable traces in sera symptom-free patients' family members, indicating a higher risk of autoimmune disease than that in general population. The careful monitoring is important to avoid not only overdiagnosis but also delay in diagnosis. Another problem is tied to sensitivity, specificity and frequency of autoantibodies—some of them are clinically significant, but observed in minority of patients, in opposite to antibodies noted in high amount of patients, but with low specificity e.g. rheumatoid factor for rheumatoid arthritis.

In gastrointestinal tract autoantibodies are indicative for autoimmune gastritis, liver diseases, biliary tract pathologies, ulcerative colitis and celiac disease. According to definition and criteria of autoimmune and autoinflammatory disease, Crohn's disease is nowadays considered to be autoinflammatory syndrome due to activation of innate immune system and lack of autoantibodies production. The autoantibodies typical for gastrointestinal diseases are shown in **Tables 1** and **2**.

Diseases and autoantibodies to	Assay	Clinical significance and comments	Comments
Celiac disease (CD)			
Tissues transglutaminase	ELISA	Highly specific, quantitative assay, diagnosis and monitoring GFD	Significant in IgA class, IgG in isolated IgA deficiency
Reticulin (endomysial)	IIF	Qualitative assay	
Atrophic gastritis (AIG)			
Parietal cells (PCA) (antigen: H+/K+ATPase)	IIF	Specific for gastritis, quantitative assay is significant for diagnosis and monitoring	Often associated with thyroid autoimmunity

Diseases and autoantibodies to	Assay	Clinical significance and comments	Comments
Intestine diseases (IBD)			
Ulcerative colitis: goblet cells (anti-mucin)	IIF	About 60% patients of UC, about 30% of Crohn's disease	Differences between regions of large bowel
pANCA (anti-MPO)	IIF	About 80% of UC patients	Present in PBC and AIH patients
Crohn's disease:			
ASCA	ELISA IIF	About 80% of Crohn's patients	Up to 25% in 1st degree relatives
Anti-pancreatic (PAB) (anti-acinar cells)	IIF	About 30% of Crohn's patients with disease localized in proximal jejunum	High specificity but low frequency

Table 1. Autoantibodies detected in serum patients with gastrointestinal disease, their clinical significance in diagnosis and differential diagnosis. *Acc.* [29, 33, 34, 38, 39, 43, 56].

Type of antibodies	Patients	Antigen	Other comments
AIH type 1:			
Antinuclear (ANA)	35–40%	Chromatin, histones, centromere, dsDNA, ssDNA, ribonucleoprotein complexes	Non-specific for AIH, seen in other autoimmune diseases
Anti-smooth muscles (SMA)	85%	Microfilaments, intermediate filaments-vimentin, desmin, polymerised F-actin	Subset of SMA, poor prognosis
Anti-actin			
Perinuclear antineutrophil antibodies (pANCA)	100%	Peripheral nuclear membrane components (pANNA), myeloperoxidase (pANCA)	pANNA specific for AIH-1 in absence of other antibodies
AIH type 2			
Liver kidney microsomal (LKMA)	100%	Cytochrome P4502D6	Present in HCV, CMV and HSV infections
Soluble liver antigen (SLA)	58–60%	O-phosphoserine tRNA, SEC tRNA syntethase	Aggressive course, relapses, poor prognosis
Liver cytosol-1 (LC-1)	60%	Formiminotransferase cyclodeaminase	Rapid progress to cirrhosis
PBC			
AMA2, 4, 8, 9	90–100%	AMA 2-inner membrane AMA 4- 8- 9-outer membrane of mitochondrium	Titre and type are not related to course of PBC
PSC			
Perinuclear antineutrophil antibodies (pANCA)	90%		Non-specific, often in patients with PSC and IBD

Table 2. Autoantibodies used for diagnosis of liver and biliary tract diseases. *Acc.* [34, 42, 44, 46, 59].

4.3. Tissue damage

In systemic autoimmune diseases, autoantibodies are playing role in tissue damage through formation of immune complexes activating classical complement cascade leading to membrane attack complex (MAC) formation. Excluding celiac disease, the role of autoantibodies in gut autoimmunity, is not fully understood, generally used as marker of process, then mechanism of tissue damage. Based on these observations, changes in tissue with irreversible damage might be described as three different components:

- First—infiltration of lymphocytes from deep crypt level to the top of villi. Flow cytometry and histochemistry analysis characterise these cells as T lymphocytes, activated T cells, B cells, plasmoblasts and plasmocytes locally producing autoantibodies. Number of intraepithelial lymphocytes (IEL) is high and infiltrating cells often formed secondary lymph nodules. Chronic inflammation is sustained by production of pro-inflammatory cytokines, and results in visible thickening of intestine wall.

- Second—presence of fibroblasts and progressing fibrotic process e.g. in liver leading to cirrhosis, in small and large ducts of biliary system leading to their walls thickening and narrowing the lumen and at the end their obstruction.

- Third—presence of other cells e.g. neutrophils, macrophages in infiltrations. These short living cells are dying within infiltrations in neighbourhood of hyper-activated adaptive immune system, what facilitates recognition of antigens and production of autoantibodies e.g. antinuclear, to myeloperoxidase (pANCA) and to others organelles. These cells produce various factors attracting new cells to come and support progression of infiltrations. They also produce variety of different trophic factors e.g.VEGF supporting neovascularisation for better nutrition of cells forming increasing infiltrations and process of fibrosis. Neutrophils form microabscesses within intestinal wall and macroabscesses between intestine loops [21–27].

Lymphocytes present in inflammation site under the epithelial layer are activated in sequential steps to develop and support chronic inflammation resulting in tissue damage. Initially, Th0 cells are activated and differentiate into different T lymphocytes functional subpopulation—Th1 with stimulation of IL-12, IL-18; Th17 with stimulation of IL-6 and TGF-β and Th2 with help of IL-4. IFN-γ and TNF, produced by Th1, activate macrophages and, in autocrine and paracrine mechanisms, stimulate further production of TNF. This activation is associated with induction of epithelial cells apoptosis and damage to first defending cellular barrier. High level of TNF facilitates maturation of stromal cells into myofibroblasts releasing metalloproteinases—tissue degrading enzymes (MMPs). IL-17 produced by Th17 is responsible for recruiting neutrophils into infiltrations during active inflammation. Even more complex and indirect is the role of IL-21, another cytokine produced by Th17, engaged in supporting of MMPs production followed by enterocyte apoptosis and basement membrane degradation [4]. In process of inflammatory infiltration formation, there is additional small subpopulation of cells with lymphocytic morphology, but without lineage determinants expression. These cells are called innate lymphoid cells (ILCs) and have ability to produce cytokines [17, 21].

5. Genetic associations of celiac disease and inflammatory bowel diseases

Observations of familiar occurrence of celiac disease indicated genetic background associated with MHC determinants. Now, this background is defined as expression of HLA-DQ2 and/or HLA-DQ8 in patients' cells. Expression of one or both of these determinants in relatives of celiac disease patient suggests introduction of diagnostic procedures for atypical (latent, late-onset) form of celiac disease [27–29]. In Crohn's disease (CD) and ulcerative colitis (UC) the genetic background was unknown until discovery of variation of NOD2 gene and IL-23 receptor gene. NOD2 is associated with severe, stricturing/penetrating course of Crohn's disease thus helps in selecting patients for more aggressive therapy. Similar association is described for DRB1*0103 and severe clinical course of UC [30, 31]. The high number of susceptibility loci discovered in Crohn's disease, now is described also for ulcerative colitis. The list of susceptibility loci for CD and UC is shown in **Table 3** with column list loci common for both diseases [30, 32]. The precise role of these loci in facilitation of development of autoimmune disease (UC) or autoinflammatory disease (CD) of gastrointestine tract is unknown. Although, the specific role of particular genes is known—genes NOD2, IIRGM, ATG16L1 in autophagy and innate immunity mediated processing of bacterias in autoinflammatory process, genes HNF4A, LAMB1, CDH1 in epithelial barrier function, see **Table 3**.

Susceptibility loci in Crohn's disease	Susceptibility loci common in Crohn's and ulcerative colitis	Susceptibility loci in ulcerative colitis
Cellular innate immunity	**Th17**	**Epithelial barrier**
NOD2, ATG16, IRGM, LRRK2	IL23R, IL12B, STAT3J, AK2, TYK2	ECM1, NHF4A, CDH1, LAMB1, GNA12
Immune-mediated	**Immune-mediated**	**Immune-mediated**
PTPN22, CCR6, IL2RA, IL18RAP, IL27, ERAP2, ITLN1, CCL2/CCL7, TNFSF11, BACH2, TAGAP, VAMP3	MST1, IL10, CARD9, REL, PRDM1, TNFSF15, ICOSLG, IL1R2, YDJC, SMAD3, PTPN2	INF□/IL26, IL8RA/IL8RB, IL2/IL21, IL7R, TNFRSF9, TNFRSF14, IRF5, LSP1
Other	**Other**	**Other**
DENNDIB, DNMT3A, GCKR, THADA, SP140, PRDX5, ZPF36L1, ZMIZ1, MUC1, CPEB4, FADS1, 5q31	NKX2-3, CREM, C11Orf30, ORMDL3, RTEL1, PTGER4, KIF21B, CDKAL1, ZNF365	OTUD3/PLA2G2E, DAP, PIM3, CAPN10
	HLA	
	DRB*103	

Table 3. List of susceptibility loci for inflammatory chronic disease of small (Crohn's disease) and large intestine (ulcerative colitis). *Acc.* [19, 30].

6. Serological diagnosis and monitoring of disease's course

The autoantibodies and antibodies in serum are detected by using indirect immunofluorescence, ELISA technique, blotting technique and radioimmune assay (RIA). In indirect immunofluorescence (IIF), the antibodies react with tissue sections and the results are visible as fluorescence of indicator tissue or cell structure (e.g. nucleus, nucleolus, centromeres, nucleus membrane proteins) after reaction with antibody. IIF helps to answer if the antibodies are present in patient's serum and what is an antigen. Semiquantitative IIF indicating titre of antibodies is based on patient's serum dilution to end-titre of positive reaction and comparison to end-titre of control serum. In case of antinuclear antibodies presence in serum, IIF is an initial step for making diagnosis. Positive result of IIF assay (end-titre higher than control) is followed by ELISA (enzyme-linked immunosorbent assay) or blotting test with eluated, precisely described antigen, e.g. dsDNA, SS-A, SS-B, Jo-1 and others associated with particular autoimmune disease, e.g. SLE, systemic sclerosis, polymyositis, neonate lupus. IIF is still used for detection of parietal cells, goblet cells antibodies, pANCA, anti-mitochondrial, LKMA and anti-smooth muscles antibodies. In ELISA, results are quantitative based on colorimetric reaction with enzyme substrate. ELISA is used for detection of antibodies to tissue transglutaminase (TTG) in diagnosis and monitoring of celiac disease, ASCA in Crohn's disease, SLA antibodies in AIH. Now, ASCA are selected from Saccharomyces cerevisiae membrane antigens—laminaribiose, chitobiose, mannobioside, laminarin, chitin and are detected in ELISA tests. The blotting technique tests are used for anti-mitochondrial antibodies type 2,4,9, antinuclear antibodies for eluated antigens detection. The RIA is last method used for antibodies detection based on counting of isotope radiation after reaction of autoantibodies with eluated antigen. This method is used for detection of antibodies circulating in low level, often below detection by above-mentioned methods, but still important for diagnosis or monitoring of disease. The typical use of RIA is detection of anti-TSH receptor antibodies in patients with thyroid diseases, autoantibodies in diabetes mellitus type 1 (GABA, insulin antibodies and others). RIA is not a common technique, because of the requirement of special isotopic laboratory. Detection of autoantibodies is generally used for diagnosis of autoimmune diseases in symptomatic individuals or in population with high risk of given disease and/or with unspecific symptoms, e.g. growth below expected, underweight, chronic diarrhoea and others typical for celiac disease. Some of antibodies are used for monitoring of therapy results—TTG antibodies in celiac patients on gluten free diet (GFD), dsDNA for SLE therapy, anti-TPO antibodies for Hashimoto disease on supplement therapy [33–46].

7. Microscopic diagnosis of inflammatory bowel diseases and celiac disease

Microscopic evaluation of mucous membrane in celiac disease, Crohn's disease and ulcerative colitis showed infiltration containing immunocompetent cells with majority of lymphoid phenotype. Biopsy is indicated for staging of villi damage in classic and atypical celiac disease, description of cellular infiltrations in Crohn's disease and ulcerative colitis. In liver diseases biopsy is essential for diagnosis and monitoring the progress of fibrosis changes leading to cirrhosis. Biopsy is usually taken during endoscopy of the upper and lower gastrointestinal tract from different parts of intestine, in majority cases from places with visible macroscopic changes. In many cases, biopsy specimens taken from normally looking mucous membrane showed the microscopic changes (infiltrations with lymphocytes and neutrophils, increased number of EIL and other), what suggested occurrence of chronic subclinical inflammatory process [24–27, 31].

8. Clinical symptoms of autoimmune diseases of gastrointestinal tract

8.1. Celiac disease

Classical celiac disease is observed in small children after introduction of gliadin, secalin or hordein (components of gluten) in diet. Typical symptoms include chronic diarrhoea, inhibition of weight gain or weight loss, abdominal pain, recurrent aphthous, changes in behaviour—'negativity', ("mister/miss no"). In delay of diagnosis the inhibition of growth, changes in enamel, low protein level lead to muscles atrophy confirmed inadequate absorption. Nowadays, this typical clinical picture is noted in no more than 15% of patients with genetically proved diagnosed celiac disease. Celiac disease may be diagnosed in any age, even in people after 50 years old. This celiac disease diagnosed later than in small children is called—latent, atypical or silent. Symptoms seen in adults are different than observed in small children. More often there are effects of defective absorption such as—anaemia due to iron deficiency, osteopenia/osteoporosis, enamel defects, aphts, (aphthous stomatitis), feeling of malaise chronic or intermittent diarrhoea, but also constipation, abdominal pain, discomfort, vomitus. Celiac disease is often associated with other autoimmune disease e.g. diabetes mellitus type 1, autoimmune thyroid diseases, autoimmune liver disease, autoimmune thrombocytopenia (mainly chronic), autoimmune Addison's disease. Moreover, celiac disease occurred about 20 times more frequently, in children with isolated IgA deficiency, CVID with low level of IgA and in about 80% of patients with dermatitis herpetiformis. Untreated celiac disease in young adults leads to unexplained subfertility, recurrent miscarriages, increasing the risk of lymphoma and gastric/large bowel carcinoma. The therapy is based on restricted gluten-free diet (GFD) [26–29, 47–50]. In humoral immunodeficiency, in about 5% of patients, the celiac disease is refractory to GFD. In refractory celiac disease (RCD), all clinical symptoms such as progressing malabsorption causing inhibition of growth, loss of weight, undernourishing, low level of vitamins, iron and proteins are observed. Moreover, introduction of immunosuppressive therapy resolves symptoms transiently or even. Patients required enteral or total parietal nutrition (TPN) for long time as supportive therapy. The use of monoclonal antibodies against TNF and/or IL-6, different combinations of immunosuppressive drugs result in partial and terminal remission in majority of patients. These patients are candidates for HSCT, even in poor clinical condition, because only this therapy offers possibility to cure the disease and save their life [51]. As alternative to HSCT from unrelated donor, autoHSCT was used for such patients with success in five out of eight patients with five-year survival in 66% [52].

8.2. Crohn's disease

Crohn's disease is lifelong disease with symptoms of chronic inflammation mediated by immune system. Like in other chronic inflammatory diseases, the inducing factor is unknown, but it is believed, that interaction between genetic background and environmental factors, mainly intestinal microbiota, leads to the disease. In last 20 years two tendencies are noted: increased number of patients and decrease in age, so children before age of 2 years fulfilling the criteria of CD are observed [19, 25, 31, 53]. The clinical symptoms are very heterogeneous, due to localization of inflammation in any part of gastrointestinal tract from mouth to anus, age of patient,

http://dx.doi.org/10.5772/67281

time of process before onset [19]. Moreover, in many patients symptoms from gastrointestinal tract are mild or unspecific, but extra-intestinal symptoms signal chronic disease. The perianal abscesses, recurrent aphthous stomatitis, fistulas, anal fissures, joints pain are noted before typical gastrointestinal symptoms like chronic or intermittens diarrhoea, pain, blood in stool and others. In young children very often the acute stage of disease is severe followed by aggressive course. Disease activity is grading as mild (Crohn's disease activity index—CDAI—150–220), moderate (CDAI—220–450) and severe (CDAI >450) [25]. Therapy is adjusted to symptoms and grading of disease at diagnosis. The antibodies to saccharomyces cerevisiae (ASCA) in IgA (and/or IgG class) are detected in high level what suggests increased intestinal barrier permeability and contact of microbiota with immunocompetent cells [19, 21, 22, 53]. Autoantibodies to acinar pancreatic cells are noted in patients with CD localized in proximal jejunum. However, the percentage of patients demonstrating these antibodies is low (about 30%), so there are not useful for diagnosis of CD. ASCA antibodies are not correlated with grading and course of disease, although, during the remission, level of ASCA is lower than in acute stage. The criterion of remission is resolving clinical symptoms up to CDAI <150 and maintenance at least for 12 months. The course of CD is unpredictable, so the remission maybe long lasting, short with relapses or chronic disease without remission. Localized disease limited to ileocaecal region only, may change into extensive disease affecting other regions in more than 100 cm in extent. In majority of patient response to steroids is very good with long remission, but in some patients, steroid-dependent form of disease or steroid-resistant form are observed. In both situations risk of accumulative side effects of steroids is high limiting prolong use of steroids, indicating introduction of second line therapy. Relapse is recognised, when symptoms are recurrent independently from therapy-maintaining remission. Diagnosis and monitoring of therapy is based on macroscopic and microscopic detection of features typical for CD. Biopsies during endoscopy are taken from involved and uninvolved areas for examination of focal or chronic inflammation, lymphocytic infiltrations, crypt irregularity, granulomas, irregular architecture of villi and other features typical for CD. In remission, biopsies from similar areas show healing of inflammation in different stages [25]. Introduction of monoclonal antibodies against TNF into therapy of CD revolutionised the therapy and medical care of CD patients, with improvement of long remission rate, comfort of live and survival of CD patients [31, 53].

8.3. Ulcerative colitis

Ulcerative colitis (UC) is a chronic inflammatory process localised exclusively in large bowel affected mucous in continuum. The course of disease is remitting and relapsing like Crohn's disease. The problem of precise diagnosis is in cases with Crohn's disease localised in large bowel overlapping clinical symptoms. Clinical symptoms in typical case of UC are associated with chronic diarrhoea, blood and mucin in stools, rectal bleeding, abdominal pain, cramps, feeling of rectal urgency and many others. The extra-intestinal symptoms are rare, present in about 10% patients with UC, as arthropathy, erythema nodosum preceding onset of typical symptoms from large bowel. In serum antibodies to pANCA are seen in about 80% of patients with typical clinical symptoms. Multiple biopsy of mucous membrane usually supports the clinical diagnosis of UC and helps in discrimination between Crohn's disease localized in large bowel and UC. Microscopic features are divided into—architectural changes, epithelial abnormalities and inflammatory features. Architectural features included crypt branching, crypt distortion, atrophy and surface irregularity. Epithelial cell abnormalities are—mucin depletion, metaplasia of Paneth cells. Inflammation is associated with infiltration lamina propria with lymphocytes, plasma cells and neutrophils, aggregates of lymphoid cells, in number of patients in lamina propria are numerous eosinophilic neutrophils. Cellular infiltrations are diffusive and transmucosal. Neutrophils migrating through crypts' epithelium are producing crypts' disruption and abscesses resulting in cell damage. Moreover, the stromal changes are associated with diffuse thickening of muscularis mucosa noted in patients with longstanding active disease or quiescent form of UC. Grading of UC is similar to Crohn's disease as mild, moderate and severe based on number of bloody stools, temperature, pulse, CRP and anaemia as result of mucous bleeding. In remission the lesions of large bowel mucous are healed and clinical symptoms resolved. Relapses are rare or frequent, in some patients are continuous without clinical and histological remission [24]. Like Crohn's disease patients are steroid-dependent or steroid-refractory, what means that therapy with steroids is not effective or effective only with high dose of steroids with risk of accumulation of side effects. Reduction of steroids dose resulted in recurrent active disease. Despite of steroid in first line 5-aminosalicylites are used but in patients with UC classified as moderate grade of disease activity. The second line of therapy included 6-mercaptopurine or azathioprine with good results in majority of patients. Good response to azathioprine or 6-mercaptopurine is associated with reduction of steroid dose what helps to avoid accumulation of side effects. Resistance to immunosuppressive therapy is indication for surgery or for biological therapy. Use of anti-TNF monoclonal antibodies gave remission in about 30% of patients. Monoclonal antibodies are used very often after surgery to prevent or reducing postoperative relapses. However, use of monoclonal antibodies, immunosuppressive therapy the rates of surgery in UC have not changed significantly [24, 54, 55]. Monoclonal antibodies used in therapy of UC are shown in **Table 4**.

8.4. Atrophic gastritis

Antibodies to parietal cells (PCA) are typical for autoimmune chronic gastritis (AIG) associated with megaloblastic anaemia in consequence of wit B12 and intrinsic factor low level due to disturbances of gastric mucous function. AIG suggested from clinical symptoms after demonstration of antibodies should be proven with gastroscopy and histological assay of mucous. Biopsy of gastric mucous is important for diagnosis of gastric cancer and premalignant stages. This wide diagnosis is important, due to prevalence of AIG in men. AIG is a progressing disease with atrophy of mucous membrane of corpus and fundus of stomach. AIG is very often noted as associated disease of thyroid autoimmune disease, diabetes type 1 in poliendocrine syndromes. In therapy, besides diet and parasols, vitamin B12 and intrinsic factor are administered parenterally with good effect in majority of patients [56, 57].

8.5. Primary biliary cirrhosis

Primary biliary cirrhosis (PBC) was the first autoimmune disease associated with jaundice and liver cirrhosis with autoantibodies in serum significant for differential diagnosis of autoimmune overlapping liver diseases. The anti-mitochondrial antibodies (AMA) are noted only in this type of biliary tract autoimmune diseases. There are typical for this type of cholangitis significant for serological diagnosis of PBC and differential diagnosis of overlapping autoimmune liver diseases [36, 58, 59]. Now, depending of antigens coming from different elements of mitochondria 9 types of AMA are described, but only AMA2, AMA4, AMA8 and AMA9 are specific for PBC and used for serological diagnosis [35, 44, 46]. ELISA technique is used for quantitative assay of AMA, but the amount of AMA is not associated with severity of symptoms and clinical course. Practically, it is enough to detect AMA2 in the serum to suggest the diagnosis of PBC [35, 59]. The study of association between MHC determinant and autoimmune disease showed the association of PBC with determinants: HLA-DR8, HLA-DR11 and HLA-DR13 in part of patients [59]. The inflammation and fibrotic process is progressing leading to cholestasis, portal fibrosis, liver cirrhosis and failure as end-stage of disease. Histological studies of biopsy showed 4 stages of PBC from portal inflammation (stage 1), through peri-portal fibrotic changes (stage 2) and bridging fibrosis (stage 3) up to symptomatic cirrhosis (stage 4) [59]. The clinical symptoms are unspecific for long time with the cholestasis as symptom of biliary ducts failure due to fibrosis followed by liver cirrhosis.

Target	Monoclonal antibody	Disease
TNF	Infliximab, Golimumab	CD, UC, RCD
	Adalimumab, Humira	CD, UC, RCD
	Certolizumab pegol	CD
	Etanercept	CD
α4-integrin	Natalizumab	CD, UC
$\alpha 4\beta 7$-integrin	Vedolizumab, Abrilumab	CD, UC
IL-12/IL-23	Ustekinumab, Briakinumab	CD
IFN-γ	Fontolizumab	CD
IL-6 receptor	Tocilizumab	CD
IL-2 receptor	Daclizumab	UC
CTLA-4	Abatacept	CD, UC
CD20	Rituximab	CD, UC, RCD
JAK1,2,3	Tofacitinib	CD
Tyrosine kinase receptor	Masitinib	CD
Anti-sense ICAM-1 inhibitor	Alicaforsen	CD

Note: CD, Crohn's disease; UC, ulcerative colitis; RCD, refractory celiac disease.

Table 4. Monoclonal antibodies used in therapy of autoimmune and autoinflammatory diseases of gastrointestinal tract and liver. *Acc.* [53].

8.6. Primary sclerosing cholangitis and autoimmune sclerosing cholangitis

The primary sclerosing cholangitis (PSC) and autoimmune sclerosing cholangitis (ASC) belong to group of biliary ducts inflammation overlapping with chronic hepatitis leading to cirrhosis. HLA-DR1 and HLA-DQ1 are often noted within patients with PSC [59]. In these diseases the anti-mitochondrial antibodies (AMA) are absent; however, the other antibodies (pANCA) are present in 60–90% of patients [46]. These antibodies are not specific for PSC, but are supporting autoimmune mechanism in PSC. The histological changes are noted in intra-hepatic and extra-hepatic biliary ducts involving small and large ducts [58]. Diffused inflammation followed with fibrosis of biliary ducts is steroid resistant in majority of patients [36]. The development of PSC and ASC is insidious and symptomless upon the moment of onset of jaundice. Patients are claiming unspecific symptoms like abdominal pain (upper right quandrant), feeling fatigue and malaise, sometimes—pruritus. PSC is a disease associated with autoimmune hepatitis but very often is a co-existent disease in ulcerative colitis and other chronic inflammatory bowel diseases. Another association of PSC is IgG4-related disease; rare clinical symptoms present in different organs, including e.g. pancreas inflammation. The immunological assays show high level of IgG4 subclass of IgG what is critical for diagnosis of basic disease. The stenosis and fibrotic changes in biliary ducts extra- and intra-hepatic, changes in liver hilar are similar to PSC and ASC. However, in IgG4-related disease the therapy based on steroids is effective, what helps to differentiate from other forms of sclerosing cholangitis [41, 45, 58–60].

8.7. Autoimmune hepatitis

Autoimmune hepatitis (AIH), chronic liver inflammation is described as AIH type-1 and AIH type-2 based on profile of autoantibodies, time of onset and response to therapy. Aetiology of autoimmune hepatitis, like other autoimmune diseases, is unknown. Moreover, the precise role of autoantibodies in given types of hepatitis, relations between types of antibodies (e.g. combination ANA/SMA), pathomechanisms leading to good response or resistance to therapy and aggressiveness of course are far from description. AIH type 1 is specified by antinuclear (ANA), anti-smooth muscles (SMA) and anti-actin antibodies. In type 2 antibodies to liver microsomal antigen (LKMA-1) and liver cells cytosol antigens (LC-1) are significant. AIH type-1 is more frequent (>80%) than AIH type-2, observed in young people (majority of patients in age below 30 years) with very good response to therapy (mostly steroids). AIH type-2 is frequently noted in children with more aggressive course, resistance to therapy with cirrhosis in about 80% of patients. The serological diagnosis is clinical significant for the estimation of therapy strategy and prognosis for patient. Some of antibodies are related to course of disease and response to therapy, e.g. anti-actin antibodies are associated with higher frequency of liver failure and patients' death, suggesting liver transplantation as life-saving procedure [59]. The presence of different profile of antibodies are seen in overlapping syndromes e.g. AIH and sclerosing cholangitis—ASC and hepatitis associated with viral infection e.g. in HCV. Difference between AIH and HCV with autoantibodies—ANA, SMA and LKMA—is histological—in HCV the tissue infiltrations containing plasma cells are absent. The occurrence of LKMA in HCV is probably the result of molecular mimicry of cytochrome 4502D6 and viral genome [46]. Another typical combination of autoimmune diseases involving liver is AIH and PBC resembled by presence of pANCA and AMA simultaneously. However, longitudinal study did not show the poorer prognosis of AIH patients with AMA compared to AIH patients without AMA in serum [46]. The combination of AIH and sclerosing cholangitis is sometimes classified as autoimmune sclerosing cholangitis—ASC [61].

Antibodies seen in AIH-1, AIH-2 and PBC are shown in **Table 2**.

8.8. Other diseases: autoimmune enteropathy

Autoimmune enteropathy (AE) is a rare disease noted in infants and young children. Clinical symptoms included severe and protracted diarrhoea followed with weight loss, malabsorption syndrome. Pathomechanism is typical for autoimmune disease with the central role of anti-epithelial antibodies. Expression of HLA class II determinants on the surface of epithelial cells in case of AE is facilitating recognition of autoantigen and stimulation of immune response with activated CD4 T lymphocytes [61]. Role of HLA class II determinants in AE was supported by observation of aberrant expression on epithelial cell from the crypts and overexpression by enterocytes suggesting local induction of autoimmune reaction with activation of intestinal T lymphocytes [62]. Clinical symptoms of AE are associated with autoimmune process against other organs and tissues. Besides autoantibodies against enterocytes, in AE antibodies toward gastric parietal cells, pancreatic islets cells, insulin, GADA, goblet cells, smooth muscles antigens, thyroid are noted. Combination of AE symptoms with autoimmune polyendocrinopathy and skin manifestation is observed in IPEX syndrome [62, 63]. In biopsy of jejunum severe villi atrophy, inflammatory infiltrations with destruction of crypt structure and depletion of goblet cells (in cases with anti-goblet cells antibodies) are observed. In majority of patients increased apoptosis of epithelial crypts is seen as typical feature [63]. Inflammatory changes are noted not only in jejunum, but in large bowel and stomach also, what indicate diffuse autoimmune disorder more difficult to control and release symptoms. Management of these patients include immunosuppression (e.g., steroids, azathioprine, cyclosporine, tacrolimus, MMF) and adequate nutritional support with correction of malabsorption effects, e.g., vitamins, calcium, proteins deficiency [62, 63]. In patients with poor response to therapy, monoclonal antibodies to TNF and immunoglobulins in high dose were introduced, but without breathtaking results. The good results on monotherapy were noted with cyclophosphamide [62].

9. Therapy of autoimmune diseases of gastrointestinal tract

9.1. Microbiota correction and diet

The use of selected bacterias for modification of dysbiosis in inflammatory bowel diseases is known from 1907 when consumption of fermented milk products containing Lactobacillus bulgaricus were used and associated with 'longevity and good health' [64]. Now, three different preparations are used—probiotics means live microorganisms with beneficial effect on host health when administered in adequate amount, prebiotics defined as selectively fermented ingredient that allows changes in composition and/or activity in gastrointestinal microflora and the last—synbiotics when probiotics and prebiotics are used simultaneously [64]. List of probiotics contains different strains of Lactobacillus, e.g., casei, rhamnosus, gasseri, Bifidobacterium, Saccharomyces boulardii and others. List of prebiotics is shorter and contains inulin, xylooligosaccharide, oligofructose and fructooligosaccharide [64, 65]. Results of probiotics, synbiotics therapy are noted as mildering course of disease (e.g., ulcerative colitis), than clinical remission or real corrections of dysbiosis [64, 65]. The effects and mechanisms of used probiotic activity in patients with IBD are shown in **Table 5**.

Antimicrobial effects	Enhancement of mucous membrane integrity	Immune modulation
Alterations in intra-intestinal environment, production antimicrobial molecules, inhibits of pathogen adhesion and cellular invasion, antitoxin effects	Increase mucous production, better epithelial barrier, changes in surface proteins	Decrease of pro-inflammatory cytokine production, increase of anti-inflammatory cytokines production, induction of Treg cells, effect on B lymphocytes
Decrease of pH in intestine lumen, production of bacteriocins, defensins, competition for adhesion sites, production of antitoxins, prevention of toxin expression	Increase function of tight junction, secretion of water and chloride	Reduction of apoptosis mediated by TNF, increase of IL-10 production, increase of secretion of IgA and production of antibodies
Prevention of Clostridium difficile infection, prevention of antibiotic-driven diarrhoea	Influence on cell-to-cell interaction, cellular stability, enhancement of epithelial cells	Prevention of antibiotic-driven diarrhoea, prevention of infectious diarrhoea, prevention of cancer

Table 5. Biological effects of probiotic, pre-biotic and synbiotic activity. *Acc.* [65].

Faecal microbial transplantation (FMT) is now a new approach to chronic microbial dysbiosis. The idea is to reintroduce and re-establish stable physiological bacterias from healthy donor supplanting dysbiotic microbiota. The first recognised successful use of this therapy was noted in patients with Clostridium difficile infection and dysbiosis in follow. In 2 weeks and 1 month after this procedure the composition of faecal bacterial containing bacterias derived mainly from donor. In spectrum of gastrointestinal disease, it seems that correction of microbiota homeostasis is indicated in Crohn's disease. According to observations and hypothesis about the role of microbial homeostasis, the bacterial dysbiosis noted in Crohn's disease is common and associated with severity of symptoms. The correction of microbiota homeostasis in these patients leads to resolving of some symptoms and help in normalisation of jejunal function [64, 66].

9.2. Classical immunosuppression

Steroids were first in autoimmune diseases therapy and up to now, there are common as first line treatment. In refractory celiac disease, autoimmune liver and biliary tract disease and IBD steroids are used to release syndromes in acute stage of disease and as maintenance therapy in remission. In CD remission was obtained with steroid in about 80% of patients in first 30 days of therapy [55]. Decrease of steroids dose, due to accumulation of side effects, is possible, when azathioprine or other classical immunosuppressant is added to therapy. Steroids are used as systemic with risk of accumulative side effects or enteral active budesonide acting in intestinal lumen with low absorption [55]. In CD, at the beginning of therapy, antibiotics were used very often, as in UC—5-aminosalicylates. Classical immunosuppression included azathioprine, methotrexate, cyclosporine A, tacrolimus and others. In children, in CD therapy, good results are obtained with cyclosporine A, but severe side effects are very often the limitation of therapy. Prolong therapy with immunosuppressant in children is resulting with inhibition of growth, puberty, cytopenias (leukopenia, neutropenia, thrombocytopenia, anaemia) and list of steroids side effects—osteopenia/osteoporosis, obesity, diabetes. Another limitation is long perspective of therapy, so accumulation of side effects is serious problem, especially for children. In UC classical immunosuppression is less effective than in CD. However, good results in UC were noted, when tacrolimus (calcineurin inhibitor) was used in therapy schedule. The target for tacrolimus and cyclosporine A is inhibition of TCR signalling, what resulted in blocking of T cell activation [14]. However, explanation why cyclosporine A is associated with good effects in CD, in opposite to UC when similar effects are obtained with tacrolimus is unknown. It maybe, that different profile of cytokines produced by given subpopulation of T lymphocytes mediating process of autoimmunity is a background for these observations. In autoimmune liver diseases steroids are used in first line of therapy together with azathioprine to reduce steroids dose and avoid side effects. In majority of AIH patients the response to this therapy in good (in about 90% of patients level of serum immunoglobulins and liver enzymes decreased to normal value). However, relapses are noted in 50–86% of patients within 6 months of remission. For these patients the second line of therapy is advice—cyclosporine A, tacrolimus, mycophenolate mofetil with success in majority of AIH patients [59].

9.3. Biological therapy

The use of monoclonal antibodies is indicated as second line of therapy after poor response to steroids and classical immunosuppression. Celiac disease is included into diseases treated with monoclonal antibodies only in the case of GFD resistance and progression of malabsorption syndrome [28, 52]. The good effect of elimination of TNF is noted only in refractory celiac disease type 1. In refractory celiac disease type 2 with T lymphocytes responsible for process and resistance to immunosuppressive therapy, infliximab is not effective. For these patients, only HSCT procedure is curative [28].

A discovery of the crucial role of TNF in regulation of pro-inflammatory cytokines production and supporting of inflammation was based on the idea of elimination of this cytokine as possible therapy. After good results observed in rheumatoid arthritis, ankylosis spondylitis patients, IBD was the next group of autoimmune diseases with successful anti-TNF therapy. In CD, anti-TNF therapy was used in refractory fistula sign form leading to surgery and disability of patients. Now, anti-TNF therapy is used in all patients with CD with indications for biological therapy, e.g. steroid refractory or steroid dependent form of disease, acute stage with severe clinical symptoms, even life-threatening, lack of remission with chronic, stable symptoms of disease. In children with CD, anti-TNF therapy is used early in disease course, often in active, severe stage, without prolonged immunosuppressive therapy carrying high risk of side effects for these patients [54, 55]. Proposition of sequential (step-by-step) therapy of CD included antibiotics and budesonide in first line, steroids and classical immunosuppression (azathioprine, methotrexate, 6-mercaptopurine) as second line and biological therapy as last line. This step-up therapy schedule maybe used as step-down after success with biological therapy, in maintaining of clinical remission. The effect of monoclonal antibodies is better, when anti-TNF antibody is used with other therapeutic, e.g., azathioprine [55]. Infliximab as anti-TNF therapy was introduced into schedule of UC therapy in 2005 year after good results of anti-TNF therapy in CD since 1998 year. Similar to CD, in UC monoclonal antibodies are used as last, third line of therapy after steroids and immunosuppression [54, 55]. In CD and UC as chronic diseases, anti-TNF therapy, like other therapy schedules, should be individualised ('patient tailored therapy'). The choice of anti-TNF antibody from, e.g., infliximab to adalimumab depends on expected effects on given symptoms of patient. The lack of effect or severe side effects contraindicated continuing therapy suggests use of monoclonal antibody against other mediator of autoimmune process, e.g., natalizumab [54]. Natalizumab is recombinant, humanised IgG4 monoclonal antibodies to α4-integrin with function of blocking this integrin. In consequence the migration of leukocytes into the intestine wall from blood is inhibited. Effect of this inhibition is noted as increase of leukocytes number in peripheral blood due to block of adhesion and transmigration out [54]. However, the fatal progressive multifocal leukoencephalopathy (PML) after natalizumab in three patients was concerned as severe side effects followed by withdrawing of this antibody from the market. Now, natalizumab is available, but for patients without other possible effective therapy [54]. Vedolizumab is used in CD and UC, but the effects of therapy are rather low. Summarising vedolizumab use is indicated in moderate-severe CD, not for UC [53]. Briakinumab was very effective in rheumatoid arthritis but without good results in CD patients. Ustekinumab as inhibitor of p40 subunit blocking IL-12 and IL-23 preventing activation of Th1, Th17 and APC (antigen presenting cells) was used with success in CD patients after anti-TNF therapy without good effect. Moreover, this antibody helps in healing of perianal symptoms of CD. Other antibodies (anti-IL-13—Dectrekumab, anti JAK inhibitors—Tofacitinib, anti-IL-6—Tocilizumab) are under clinical trials and pilot studies [53].

New promising biological therapies are directed against different molecules, including cytokines produced by autoreactive T lymphocytes mediating chronic inflammation. Monoclonal antibodies against interleukins, interleukins receptors, integrins, IFN are used in different clinical trials in CD and UC [54]. List of antibodies used in biological therapy is shown in **Table 4**.

9.4. Haematopoietic stem cell transplantation procedure

In celiac disease and IBD indications of HSCT procedure are associated with co-existent disease, e.g., haematological or severe course, resistant to therapy or diet with progression of malabsorption syndrome. Decision of HSCT is difficult, because patients resistant to therapy with progress of disease, are usually on total parietal nutrition, with recurrent, prolong or opportunistic infections, malabsorption syndrome with high risk of death after HSCT procedure. Another therapy proposed is mesenchymal cell application (MSC)—used intraperitoneally, intravenously. However, the results are not conclusive, although a decrease of pro-inflammatory cytokines in mucous biopsy was noted [51, 52].

10. Conclusions

Certain gastrointestinal tract diseases are classified as autoinflammatory/autoimmune due to chronic course with remissions and exacerbations, histological and serological features, good response to immunosuppressive treatment. Therapy is based on inhibition of immune system activation, reduction of inflammatory process, decrease of antibody production and complexes formation. Steroids are commonly used to obtain and, in small doses, to maintain remission. However, severe side effects or steroid resistance implicate the usage of classical immunosuppressive drugs. Classification of gastrointestinal tract diseases as autoimmune opened the opportunity for analogical treatment with other autoimmune diseases including monoclonal antibodies. Moreover, for progressive cases with poor prognosis haematopoietic stem cell, transplantation is proposed with encouraging results.

Author details

Anna Pituch-Noworolska* and Monika Mach-Tomalska

*Address all correspondence to: mipituch@cyf-kr.edu.pl

Department of Clinical Immunology, Institute of Pediatrics, Medical College, Jagiellonian University, Kraków, Poland

References

[1] Leone VA., Cham CM., Chang EB.: Diet, gut and genetics in immune function. Curr. Opin. Immunol. 2014, 0, 16–23, doi:10.1016/j.coi.014.08.004.

[2] Littman DR., Pamer EG.: Role of commensal microbiota in normal and pathogenic host immune response. Cell Host Microbe. 2011, 10, 311–323.

[3] Elson ChO., Alexander KL.: Host-microbiota interactions in the intestine. Dig. Dis. 2015, 33, 131–136.

[4] Geremia A., Biancheri P., Allan Ph., Corazza GR., Di Sabatino A.: Innate and adaptive immunity in inflammatory bowel disease. Autoimmunity Rev. 2014, 13, 3–10.

[5] Kurashima Y., Goto Y., Kiyono H.: Mucosal innate immune cells regulate both Gut homeostasis and intestinal inflammation. Eur. J. Immunol., 2013, 43, 3108–3115.

[6] Shaw PJ., McDermott MF., Kanneganti T-D.: Inflammasomes and autoimmunity. Trends Mol. Med. 2011, 17, 57–64.

[7] Kayama H., Takeda K.: Regulation of intestinal homeostasis by innate and adaptive immunity. Internat. Immunol. 2012, 24, 673–680.

[8] Kato LM., Kawamoto S., Maruya M., Fagarasan S.: The role of adaptive immune system in regulation of gut microbiota. Immunol. Rev. 2014, 260, 67–75.

[9] Reboldi A., Arnon TI., Rodda LB., Atakilit A., Sheppard D., Cyster JG.: IgA production requires B cell interaction with subepithelial dendritic cells in Peyer's patches. Science, 2016, 352, aaf4822-1-aaf4822-7

[10] Xiong N., Hu Sh.: Regulation of intestinal IgA responses. Cell Mol. Life Sci. 2015, 72, 2645–2655.

[11] Doria A, Zen M., Bettio S., Gatto M., Bassi N., Nalotto L., Ghirardello A., Iaccarino L., Punzi L.: Autoinflammation and autoimmunity. Autoimmunity Rev. 2012, 12, 22–30.

[12] Hedrich ChD.: Shaping the spectrum – from autoinflammation to autoimmunity. Clin. Immunol. 2016, 165, 21–28.

[13] Wilson SP., Cassel SL.: Inflammasome mediated autoinflammatory disorders. Postgrad. Med., 2010, 122, 125–133.

[14] Steward-Tharp SM., Song Y-j., Siegel RM., O'Shea JJ.: New insights into T cell biology and T-cell directed therapy for autoimmunity, inflammation and immunosuppression. Ann. N.Y. Acad. Sci 2010, 1183, 123–148.

[15] Balague C., Kunkel SL., Godessart N.: Understanding autoimmune disease. Drug Discov. Today 2009, 14, 926–934.

[16] Galiani N., Huber S.: Balancing pro-and anti-inflammatory CD4+ T helper cells in the intestine. In:" Autoimmune Diseases" *edited by J. Chan, ISBN 978-953-51-0693-7, Published: July 25, 2012 , pp. 51–76.*

[17] Wallace KL., Zheng L-B., Kanazawa Y., Shih DQ.: Immunopathology of inflammatory bowel disease. World J. Gastroenterol. 2014, 20, 6–21.

[18] El-Khider F., McDonald Ch.: Links of autophagy dysfunction to inflammatory bowel disease onset. Dig. Dis. 2016, 34, 27–34.

[19] Marcuzzi A., Bianco AM., Girardelli M., Tommasini A., Martelossi S., Manosta L., Crovella S.: Genetic and functional profiling of Crohn's disease: autophagy mechanisms and susceptibility to infectious diseases. BioMed. Res. Intern. 2013, Article ID 297501, 1–11.

[20] Elkon K., Casali P.: Nature and function of autoantibodies. Nat. Clin. Pract. Rheumatol. 2006, 4, 491–498.

[21] Abdullah M., Syam AF., Simadibrata M., Dunawan J., Makmun D., Rani AA.: New insight on the pathomechanisms of inflammatory bowel disease. J. Dig. Dis. 2013, 14, 455–462.

[22] Kaser A., Zeissig S., Blimberg RS.: Inflammatory bowel disease. Annu. Rev. Immunol. 2010, 28, 573 – 621.

[23] Kim YS., Ho SB.: Intestinal goblet cells and mucin in health and disease. Curr. Gastroenterol. Rep. 2010, 12, 3190330.

[24] Stange EF., Travis SPL., Vermeire S., Reinisch W.,Geboes K., Barakauskiene A., Feakins R., Flejou JF., Herfarth H., Hommes DW., Kupcinskas L., Lakatros PL., Mantzaris GJ., Schreiber S., Villanacci V., Warren BF.: European evidence-based consensus on the diagnosis and management of ulcerative colitis. J. Crohn Colitis 2008, 2, 1–23.

[25] Stange EF., Travis SPL., Vermeire S., Berlinger C., Kupcinskas L., Geboes K., Barakauskiene A., Villanacci V., von Herbay A., Warren BF., Gasche C., Tilg H., Schreiber SW., Scholmerich J., Reinisch W.: European evidence-based consensus on the diagnosis and management of Crohn'd disease. Gut 2006, 55, i1–i15.

[26] Sbarbati A., Valletta E., Bertini M., Cipolli M., Morroni M., Pinelli L., Tato l.: Gluten sensitivity and "normal' histology. Dig. Liver Dis. 2003, 35, 768–773.

[27] Walker M., Murray JA.: An update in the diagnosis of celiac disease. Histopathology 2011, 59, 166–179.

[28] Al-toma A., Verbeek WHM., Mulder CJJ.: The management of complicated celiac disease. Dig. Dis. 2007, 25, 230–236.

[29] Torres MI., Palomeque T., Lorite P.: Celiac disease and other autoimmune disorders. In:"Autoimmunity-Pathogenesis, clinical aspects and therapy of sepecific autoimmune diseases", *edited by K. Chatzidionysiou, ISBN 978-953-51-2134-3, Published: June 17, 2015,* pp. 131–151.

[30] Lees CW., Barrett JC., Parkes M., Satsangi J.: New IBD genetics. Gut 2011, 60, 1739–1753.

[31] Schirbel A., Fiocchi C.: Inflammatory bowel disease. J. Dig. Dis. 2010, 1, 266–276.

[32] Uhlig HH.: Monogenic diseases associated with intestinal inflammation. Gut 2013, 62, 1795–1805.

[33] Ardesjo B., Portela-Gomes GM., Rorsman F., Gerdin E., Loof L., Grimelius L., Kampe O., Ekwall O.: Immunoreactivity against goblet cells in patients with inflammatory bowel disease. Inflamm. Bowel Dis. 2008, 5, 652–661.

[34] Bogdanos DP., Invernizzi P., Mackay IR., Vergani D.: Autoimmune liver serology. World J. Gastroenterol. 2008, 14, 3374–3387.

[35] Bogdanos DP., Rigopoulou EI., Smyk DS., Roggenbuck D.,Reinhold D., Forbes A., Laass MW., Cobrad K.: Diagnostic value, clinical utility and pathogenic significance of reactivity to the molecular targets of Crohn's disease specific-pancreatic autoantibodies. Autoimmun. Rev. 2011, 11, 143–148.

[36] Grant C.R., Liberal R.: Liver immunology:How to reconcile tolerance with autoimmunity. Clin. Res. Hepatol. Gastroenterol. 2017;41:6-16

[37] Invernizzi P., Mackay IR.: Autoimmune liver serology. World J. Gastroenterol. 2008, 14, 3374–3387.

[38] Kuna AT.: Serological markers of inflammatory bowel disease. Biochemia Med. 2013, 23, 28–42.

[39] Lidnfors K., Kaukinen K.: Contribution of celiac disease autoantibodies to the disease process. Expert Rev. Clin. Immunol. 2012, 8, 151–154.

[40] Liberal R., Mieli-Vergani G., Vergani D.: Clinical significance of autoantibodies in autoimmune hepatitis. J. Autoimmunity 2013, 46, 17–24.

[41] Lee SP., Roberts JR., Kuver R.: The changing faces of cholangitis. F1000Research 2016, 1409, 1–7.

[42] Makol A., Watt KD., Chowdhary VR.: Autoimmune hepatitis. Hepat. Res. Treat. 2011, Article ID 390916, 1–11.

[43] Papp M., Norman GL., Altorjay I., Lakatos PL.: Utility of serological markers in inflammatory bowel diseases: gadget or magic? World J. Gastroenterol. 207, 13, 2028–2036.

[44] Sener AG.: Autoantibodies in liver diseases. APMIS 2015, 123, 915–919.

[45] Zen Y., Kawakami H., Kim JH.: IgG4-related sclerosing cholangitis: All we need to know. J. Gastroenterol. 2016, 51, 295–312.

[46] Zeman MV., Hirschfield GM.: Autoantibodies and liver diseases. Can. J. Gastroenterol. 2010, 24, 225–231.

[47] Barton SH., Murray JA.: Celiac disease and autoimmunity in the gut and elsewhere. Gastroenterol. Clin. North Am. 2008, 37, 411–428.

[48] Nejad MR., Rostami K., Pourhoseingholi MA., Mojarad EN., Habibi M., Dabiri H., Zali MR.: Atypical presetation is dominant and typical for coeliac disease. J. Gastrointestin. Liver Dis. 2009, 18, 285–291.

[49] Troncone R., Discepolo V.: Celiac disease and autoimmunity. JPGN. 2014, 59 Suppl. 1, S9–S11.

[50] Pituch-Noworolska A., Zwonarz K.: Celiac and inflammatory bowel diseases in children with primary humoral immunodeficiency. In: "Autoimmunity-Pathogenesis, clinical aspects and therapy of specific autoimmune diseases", *edited by K. Chatzidionysiou, ISBN 978-953-51-2134-3, Published June 17, 2015*, pp. 151–172.

[51] Ciccocioppo R., Cangemi GC., Kruzliak P., Corazza GR.: Concise review: Cellular therapies: The potential to regenerate and restore tolerance in immune-mediated intestinal diseases. Stem Cells 2016;34(6): 1474–86.

[52] Nijeboer P., van Wanrooij RLJ., Tack GJ., Mulder CJJ., Bouma G.: Update on the diagnosis and management of refractory celiac disease. Gastroenterol. Res. Pract. 2013, Article ID 516 483 pp. 1–9.

[53] Manuc T-E., Manuc MM., Diculescu MM.: Recent insight into the molecular pathogenesis of Crohn's disease: a review of emerging therapeutic targets. Clin. Exp. Gastroeneterol. 2016, 9, 59–70.

[54] Rutgeerts PL., Vermeire S., van Assche G.: Biological therapies for inflammatory bowel diseases. Gastroenterol. 2009, 136, 1182–1197.

[55] Valeyos FS., Sandborn WJ.: Positioning biologic therapy for Crohn's disease and ulcerative colitis. Current Gastroenterol. Rep. 2007, 9, 521–527.

[56] Tozzoli R., Kadermaz G., Perosa AR., Tampoia M., Zucano A., Antico A., Bizzaro N.: Autoantibodies to parietal cells as predictors of atrophic gastritis. Autoimmunity Rev. 2010, 10, 80–83.

[57] Weck MN., Brenner H.: Prevalence of chronic atrophic gastritis in different parts of the world. Cancer Epidemiol. Biomarkers Prev. 2006, 15, 1083–1094.

[58] Czaja AJ.: The overlap syndromes of autoimmune hepatitis. Dig. Dis. Sci. 2013, 58, 326–343.

[59] Czaja AJ.: Diagnosis and management of autoimmune hepatitis. Gut Liver 2016, 10, 177–203.

[60] Than NN., Oo YH.: A concise review of autoimmune liver diseases. in:"Autoimmunity Pathogenesis, clinical aspects and therapy of specific autoimmune diseases", *edited by K. Chatzidionysiou, ISBN 978-953-51-2134-3, Published: June 17, 2015*, pp. 97–130.

[61] Mieli-Vergani G., Vergani D.: Autoimmune paediatric liver disease. World J. Gastroenterol. 2008, 14, 3360–3367.

[62] Montalto M., D'Onofrio F., Santoro L., Gallo A., Gasbarrini A., Gasborrini G.: Autoimmune enteropathy in children and adults. Scand. J. Gastroenterol. 2009, 44, 1029–1036.

[63] Russo P., Alvarez F.: Autoimmune enteropathy. Clin. Appl. Immunol. Rev. 2002, 2, 203–216.

[64] Bull MJ., Plummer NT.: Treatments for chronic gastrointestinal disease and gut dysbiosis. Integr. Med. 2015, 14, 25–33.

[65] Patel R., DuPont HL.: New approaches for bacteriotherapy: prebiotics, new-generation probiotics, and synbiotics. Clin. Infect. Dis. 2015, 60, S106–S121.

[66] Lopez J., Grinspan A.: Faecal microbiots transplantation for inflammatory bowel disease. Gastroenterol. Hepatol. 2016, 12, 374–379.

Chapter 6

Translating Autoimmune Pathogenesis into Targeted Therapies for Systemic Sclerosis

Mark D. Russell and Nidhi Sofat

Additional information is available at the end of the chapter

http://dx.doi.org/10.5772/66642

Abstract

Targeted therapies including tumour necrosis factor α (TNFα) inhibitors have transformed the management of a number of autoimmune conditions over the past 20 years. One autoimmune rheumatological condition with significant potential for the development of targeted therapies is systemic sclerosis (SSc). In this chapter, we use SSc as an example of how research into the pathogenic processes underlying autoimmune conditions can be translated into novel targeted therapies. We review the evidence base for a range of targeted therapies for SSc identified from a systematic literature search, before highlighting a number of studies currently underway.

Keywords: systemic sclerosis, scleroderma, targeted therapies, biological therapy, biologic, rheumatology, rheumatoid arthritis, autoimmune

1. Introduction

1.1. Targeted therapies in autoimmune conditions

Targeted therapies have revolutionised the management of many autoimmune rheumatological conditions over the last 20 years. Ground-breaking research in the early 1990s identified tumour necrosis factor alpha (TNFα) as a key inflammatory mediator of rheumatoid arthritis [1–6]. This research enabled the development of targeted TNFα inhibitors, such as adalimumab, infliximab and etanercept. Although costly, these therapies have greatly improved the outlook for patients with severe, active rheumatoid arthritis [7, 8].

As we improve our understanding of the pathogenic processes underlying rheumatoid arthritis, the number of potential targets for novel therapies increases. Several additional targeted therapies are now licensed for the treatment of patients with severe rheumatoid arthritis who have failed to respond adequately to, or been unable to tolerate, conventional immunosuppressive therapies. Examples include: rituximab, a B-lymphocyte-depleting monoclonal antibody targeting the CD20 antigen; abatacept, a fusion protein that abrogates the co-stimulatory signals required for the activation of T-lymphocytes; tocilizumab, an interleukin (IL)-6 receptor antagonist; and anakinra, an IL-1 receptor antagonist [8–13].

The process of translating research on autoimmune pathogenesis into targeted therapies has not been limited to rheumatoid arthritis, however. TNFα inhibitors have also been shown to be highly effective in psoriasis and psoriatic arthritis, as well as ankylosing spondylitis, juvenile idiopathic arthritis and inflammatory bowel disease [14–17]. Targeted therapies with novel mechanisms of action have also been developed for a number of autoimmune rheumatological conditions. Ustekinumab, a humanised monoclonal antibody directed against IL-12/23, is licensed as a treatment for both psoriasis and psoriatic arthritis [18]. Secukinumab, an IL-17 inhibitor, has also been shown to be efficacious in the treatment of both psoriasis and psoriatic arthritis [19, 20]. In the case of autoantibody-positive systemic lupus erythematosus, belimumab, an inhibitor of B-lymphocyte stimulator, has recently been licensed as an adjunctive therapy [21].

An autoimmune rheumatological condition with a great need for targeted therapies is systemic sclerosis (SSc). In this chapter, we use SSc as an example of how research into pathogenic processes can be translated into novel therapeutic targets for autoimmune conditions.

1.2. Background to systemic sclerosis

SSc is a multi-system autoimmune condition that typically arises between the ages of 30 and 50 years, with women affected approximately four times more frequently than men. The aetiology of SSc remains to be elucidated and is likely to involve complex interactions between environmental factors in genetically predisposed individuals. Multiple cell types, cytokines and signalling pathways contribute to three sustained and interdependent pathogenic processes that form the hallmark of SSc: excessive extracellular matrix production and deposition by fibroblasts, inflammation and vascular abnormalities [22]. These processes culminate in multi-organ fibrosis, in addition to vascular manifestations, such as pulmonary arterial hypertension (PAH), Raynaud's phenomenon (RP) and renal crises.

Fibrotic thickening and hardening of the skin, termed sclerodactyly, can lead to profound physical and psychological morbidity. Gastrointestinal tract fibrosis can produce a range of complications depending on the portions of the tract involved, including oesophageal reflux and strictures, gastroparesis, small bowel bacterial overgrowth and constipation. Pulmonary involvement represents the leading cause of death in patients with SSc, with interstitial lung disease (ILD) and PAH typically presenting with progressive breathlessness on exertion. Two additional presenting features of SSc, often occurring in the early stages of the disease, are digital swelling and RP. In the case of the latter, vasospastic changes produce a characteristic whitening of the distal portions of the fingers and toes that progresses to a blue discolouration (representing cyanosis), before flushing red as blood flow returns. In SSc, RP can be severe enough to result in digital ulceration and necrosis.

http://dx.doi.org/10.5772/66642

SSc can be subdivided into two main forms depending on the extent of skin involvement. In limited cutaneous systemic sclerosis (lcSSc), fibrosis occurs in the skin of the face and in the skin distal to the elbows and knees. A term often used interchangeably with lcSSc is CREST syndrome, an acronym representing five cardinal signs and symptoms that arise in a subset of patients with lcSSc: calcinosis, RP, oesophageal dysmotility, sclerodactyly and telangiectasia. Diffuse cutaneous systemic sclerosis (dcSSc) is characterised by more extensive skin involvement than lcSSc, such that the proximal arms, legs and trunk are often affected. The onset and progression of skin changes are usually more rapid in dcSSc than in lcSSc, with multi-organ fibrosis typically occurring to a greater extent.

1.3. Management of systemic sclerosis

The mainstay of management of SSc involves close monitoring for systemic complications, with treatment as they arise [22]. A multidisciplinary approach is essential, with involvement of clinicians from a range of specialties, as well as physiotherapists, occupational therapists and psychologists [23, 24].

For skin involvement, topical steroids and emollients can help to ameliorate any associated pruritus and xerosis. Camouflage products are also effective in minimising the cosmetic effects of hypopigmented and hyperpigmented areas of skin, as well as telangiectasia. Regular physiotherapy, along with orthoses, decreases the risk of sclerodactyly-induced contractures. However, surgery may ultimately be required in the case of established contractures.

Acid-suppressant therapies, such as proton-pump inhibitors, and pro-motility agents, such as metoclopramide, are frequently used to treat SSc-associated gastro-oesophageal reflux and gastroparesis, respectively. Should strictures of the oesophagus arise, endoscopic dilatation can be employed. With more distal gastrointestinal tract involvement, dietetic input can help to counter the malabsorptive effects of small bowel dysmotility and bacterial overgrowth. The latter may also necessitate cyclical treatment with antibiotics. Laxative therapy, pro-motility agents and ensuring an adequate intake of fibre can minimise the constipation that arises from colonic dysmotility.

A potentially fatal complication of SSc, requiring emergent treatment, is a scleroderma renal crisis. This typically presents with acute-onset hypertension and renal impairment, and can rapidly progress to renal failure without prompt recognition and treatment. Angiotensin-converting enzyme inhibitors are the cornerstone of management of such crises. Their use has greatly improved the prognosis associated with scleroderma renal crises, such that this complication is no longer the leading cause of death in patients with systemic sclerosis.

Significant progress has also been made in the management of SSc-associated RP. Treatment options available include calcium-channel blockers, such as nifedipine, phosphodiesterase type-5 inhibitors, such as sildenafil, and angiotensin II receptor antagonists, such as losartan. In cases of digital ulceration and impending digital necrosis, inpatient admission may be required for intravenous prostanoid therapy. Phosphodiesterase type-5 inhibitors and prostaglandin infusions are also effective treatments for SSc-associated PAH. Additionally, bosentan, an endothelin-receptor antagonist, has been shown to be efficacious in the management of both SSc-associated PAH and digital ulcers. Bosentan is a rare example of a targeted therapy licensed for use in SSc and is covered in greater detail later in this chapter.

Multiple immunosuppressive medications have been trialled in SSc. The evidence base is weak, however, and clinical trials of such medications are limited by the rarity and heterogeneity of SSc, and the variability in the natural progression of the disease. As is true of other autoimmune rheumatological conditions, there is a growing trend for early, aggressive treatment of SSc with immunosuppressive regimens [23, 24]. This is particularly true of dcSSc, where early immunosuppression has the potential to stem the progression of the disease. Typical first-line treatment options for SSc-associated ILD include intravenous cyclophosphamide (as induction therapy) followed by an oral agent such as mycophenolate mofetil (as maintenance therapy). In cases of extensive SSc-associated skin fibrosis, treatment options include mycophenolate mofetil and methotrexate, as well as azathioprine, cyclophosphamide and corticosteroid therapy [24].

Relative to other autoimmune conditions, such as rheumatoid arthritis, the efficacy of immunosuppressive regimens in the treatment of SSc is modest [25]. Broad-spectrum immunosuppression also carries with it the risk of infection and bone marrow suppression, as well as agent-specific side effects, such as bladder toxicity with cyclophosphamide therapy. As such, there is a concerted effort to find novel treatment options for SSc. One example is autologous haematopoietic stem cell transplantation, which has a growing evidence base in SSc. In selected patients with early dcSSc and poor prognostic features, stem cell transplantation has been shown to improve long-term event-free and overall survival rates, relative to IV cyclophosphamide [26, 27]. These benefits have to be weighed against early transplant-related mortality rates of 10%, however. As such, the use of stem cell transplantation is restricted to those patients with early dcSSc who are yet to develop severe organ involvement. Another example of an emerging therapy is intravenous immunoglobulin (IVIg), with a number of pilot studies reporting improvements in skin fibrosis scores, gastrointestinal manifestations and joint-related symptoms [28–31].

Despite some progress in the management of SSc, there remains a great need for therapies that target the specific pathogenic processes underlying the disease, namely fibrosis, inflammation and vascular damage. The development of efficacious targeted therapies has the potential to transform the management of this disabling condition, just as TNFα inhibitors have done in rheumatoid arthritis, psoriatic arthritis and ankylosing spondylitis. In this chapter, we use SSc as an example of how research into pathogenic processes can be translated into novel therapeutic targets for autoimmune conditions.

2. Body

We performed a systematic search of the PubMed and Cochrane medical literature databases to identify all clinical studies involving therapeutic interventions in patients with systemic sclerosis during the last 10 years (covering the period of July 2006–June 2016). Using a broad search strategy, we identified 2381 articles. We reviewed the abstracts of these articles and

http://dx.doi.org/10.5772/66642

selected those studies involving therapies with targeted mechanisms of action, that is, treatments targeting specific molecular and/or cellular pathways known to be involved in the pathogenesis of SSc. Studies were excluded if they were not written in English, if they did not involve human subjects or if they had less than three study subjects. In total, 69 studies were identified and the details are shown in **Table 1**. The majority of the therapies identified can be grouped into three broad categories, corresponding to which of the central pathogenic processes they target: fibrosis, inflammation or vascular abnormalities. It is important to note, however, that these processes are very much interdependent and, as such, targeting one pathway is likely to impact on one or more of the other processes [32].

Study treatment	Ref.	Treatment dosage	Disease aspect studied	Study type	Duration of study	Number drug/ control	*p*-value (measure)
Fibrosis							
TGF-β pathway inhibitors							
CAT-192	[35]	Various	dcSSc	RCT	6 months	32/11	>0.05 (mRSS)
Fresolimumab	[37]	Various	dcSSc	Prospective	24 weeks	15/0	<0.001 (mRSS)
Pirfenidone	[42]	2403 mg daily	SSc-ILD	Prospective	16 weeks	63/0	>0.05 (PFTs, mRSS)
Pirfenidone	[43]	1200/1800 mg daily	SSc-ILD	Case series	Various	5/0	N/A
Tyrosine kinase inhibitors							
Imatinib mesylate	[45]	400 mg daily	dcSSc	RCT	6 months	9/1	>0.05 (mRSS)
Imatinib mesylate	[46]	600 mg daily	SSc-ILD	Prospective	12 months	20/0	>0.05 (PFTs), <0.001 (mRSS)
Imatinib mesylate	[47]	400 mg daily	dcSSc	Prospective	12 months	30/0	<0.001 (mRSS), 0.008 (FVC)
Imatinib mesylate	[48]	400 mg daily	dcSSc	Prospective	36 months	17/0	0.002 (mRSS)
Imatinib mesylate	[49]	200 mg daily	SSc-ILD	Prospective	12 months	30/0	N/A
Imatinib mesylate	[126]	400 mg daily	SSc/ morphoea	RCT	12 months	15/13	>0.05 (mRSS)
Imatinib mesylate	[127]	200 mg daily	SSc	Case series	23 months	6/0	N/A
Imatinib mesylate	[128]	100 mg daily	SSc skin	Case series	6 months	3/0	N/A
Imatinib mesylate + CYC	[129]	200 mg daily	SSc-ILD	Case series	12 months	5/0	N/A
Nilotinib	[50]	800 mg daily	dcSSc	Prospective	12 months	10/0	0.02 (mRSS)
Other agents							

Study treatment	Ref.	Treatment dosage	Disease aspect studied	Study type	Duration of study	Number drug/ control	*p*-value (measure)
Oral type I collagen	[51]	500 μg daily	dcSSc	RCT	15 months	83/85	>0.05 (mRSS)
Relaxin	[53]	10/25 μg/kg daily	dcSSc	RCT	24 weeks	137/94	>0.05 (mRSS)
Inflammation							
TNFα inhibitors							
TNFα inhibitors	[54]	Various	SSc	Retrospective	Various	65/0	N/A
Etanercept	[60]	50 mg/week	SSc-m'skel	Retrospective	Various	18/0	>0.05 (HAQ, mRSS)
Infliximab	[61]	5 mg/kg ×5	dcSSc	Prospective	26 weeks	16/0	>0.05 (mRSS, HAQ)
Selective co-stimulation modulators							
Abatacept	[67]	500/1000 mg ×7	dcSSc	RCT	24 weeks	7/3	0.06 (mRSS)
Abatacept + tocilizumab	[68]	Various	SSc-m'skel	Observational	11 months	27/0	<0.001 (DAS28)
Abatacept	[130]	500/750 mg/4 weeks	dcSSc	Case series	Various	4/0	N/A
IL-2α inhibitors							
Basiliximab	[72]	20 mg ×6	dcSSc	Prospective	68 weeks	10/0	0.015 (mRSS), >0.05 (FVC/DLco)
IL-6 inhibitors							
Tocilizumab + abatacept	[68]	Various	SSc-m'skel	Observational	5 months	27/0	0.001 (DAS28)
Tocilizumab	[77]	8 mg/kg/4 weeks	SSc	Case series	Various	3/0	N/A
Tocilizumab	[78]	162 mg/week	SSc	RCT	48 weeks	43/44	0.09 (mRSS)
B-cell depletion							
Rituximab	[81]	Various	SSc	Case-control	Various	63/25	0.03 (mRSS), 0.02 (FVC)
Rituximab	[82]	1000 mg ×2	dcSSc	Prospective	6 months	15/0	>0.05 (mRSS)
Rituximab	[83]	(500 mg ×2)/3 months	SSc-ILD	Case series	12 months	5/0	<0.001 (mRSS, DLco), <0.004 (FVC)
Rituximab	[84]	1000 mg ×2	dcSSc	Prospective	24 weeks	8/0	<0.001 (mRSS)
Rituximab	[85]	1000 mg ×2	SSc	Prospective	36 months	9/0	0.001 (mRSS)

Study treatment	Ref.	Treatment dosage	Disease aspect studied	Study type	Duration of study	Number drug/ control	p-value (measure)
Rituximab	[86]	(375 mg/m^2 ×4)/6 months	dcSSc	Prospective	12 months	25/0	0.001 (FVC), 0.008 (DLco), 0.0001 (mRSS)
Rituximab	[87]	(375 mg/m^2 ×4)/24 weeks	SSc	RCT	12 months	8/6	0.002 (FVC), <0.001 (mRSS)
Rituximab	[88]	(375 mg/m^2 ×4)/6 months	SSc-ILD	Prospective	24 months	8/0	<0.0001 (FVC, mRSS), <0.001 (DLco)
Rituximab	[89]	(1000 mg ×2)/6 months	dcSSc	Prospective	24 months	8/0	<0.0001 (mRSS, DAS)
Rituximab	[90]	Various	SSc	Prospective	7 years	30/0	0.018 (FVC), 0.012 (DLco), <0.001 (mRSS)
MEDI-551	[91]	Various	SSc	RCT	85 days	24/4	N/A
Type I IFN receptor antagonists							
MEDI-546	[92]	Various	SSc	Prospective	12 weeks	34/0	N/A
Vascular							
Endothelin receptor antagonists							
Bosentan	[97]	250 mg daily	SSc-RP/skin	Retrospective	48 weeks	14/0	<0.05 (RP attacks), <0.01 (mRSS)
Bosentan	[99]	250 mg daily	SSc-PAH	Prospective	Various	49/0	0.014 (NYHA class), >0.05 (6MWD)
Bosentan	[100]	250 mg daily	SSc-DU	RCT	24 weeks	98/90	0.04 (DU episodes), >0.05 (DU healing)
Bosentan	[101]	250 mg daily	SSc-DU	Retrospective	24 months	67/0	N/A
Bosentan	[102]	250 mg daily	SSc-DU	Prospective	36 months	26/0	<0.001 (DU number)
Bosentan	[103]	62.5–125 mg daily	SSc-DU	Case series	Various	6/0	N/A
Bosentan	[108]	250 mg daily	SSc-RP	Prospective	16 weeks	15/0	<0.05 (RP attacks)
Bosentan	[112]	250 mg daily	SSc-ILD	RCT	12 months	77/86	>0.05 (6MWD, PFTs)
Bosentan	[113]	250 mg daily	SSc-ILD	Prospective	24 months	9/0	N/A

Study treatment	Ref.	Treatment dosage	Disease aspect studied	Study type	Duration of study	Number drug/ control	*p*-value (measure)
Bosentan	[114]	250 mg daily	SSc-skin	Prospective	24 weeks	10/0	<0.001 (mRSS, DU healing)
Bosentan + iloprost	[131]	250 mg daily	SSc-vascular	Observational	3 years	13/13	<0.01 (PBP)
Bosentan	[132]	250 mg daily	SSc-DU/PAH	Prospective	Various	54/0	<0.001 (DU episodes)
Bosentan	[133]	250 mg daily	SSc-NDU	Case series	Various	5/0	N/A
Bosentan	[134]	250 mg daily	SSc-vascular	Prospective	16 weeks	30/30	N/A
Bosentan	[135]	250 mg daily	SSc-RP	RCT	24 weeks	9/8	>0.05 (RP attacks), 0.01 (HAQ)
Bosentan	[136]	250 mg daily	CTD-PAH/ skin	Observational	24 months	15/0	<0.01 (6MWD, mRSS),
Bosentan	[137]	250 mg daily	CTD-PAH	Prospective	48 weeks	53/0	N/A
Bosentan	[138]	250 mg daily	SSc-DU	Prospective	Various	15/0	<0.05 (DU number)
Bosentan	[139]	125 mg daily	SSc-vascular	Prospective	4 weeks	12/12	<0.001 (FMD)
Bosentan	[140]	250 mg daily	SSc-vascular	Prospective	6 months	18/0	>0.05 (multiple measures)
Bosentan	[141]	250 mg daily	SSc-RP	Observational	16 weeks	3/0	N/A
Bosentan	[142]	250 mg daily	SSc-PAH	Prospective	6 months	8/0	0.01 (6MWD)
Bosentan	[143]	250 mg daily	SSc-DU	Prospective	12 weeks	52/51	<0.05 (blood flow)
Bosentan	[144]	250–500 mg daily	CTD-PAH	RCT	12-16 weeks	44/22	>0.05 (6MWD)
Ambrisentan + tadalafil	[105]	10 + 40 mg	SSc-PAH	Prospective	36 weeks	24/0	<0.05 (RV mass), <0.0001 (PVR)
Ambrisentan	[106]	5–10 mg daily	SSc-PAH	Prospective	24 weeks	12/0	0.004 (PVR), 0.003 (6MWD)
Ambrisentan	[107]	5 mg daily	SSc-DU/RP	Prospective	6 months	6/0	<0.03 (DU healing), 0.01 (RP attacks)
Ambrisentan	[145]	Up to 10 mg/day	SSc-DU	Prospective	24 weeks	20/0	0.004 (DU number)/0.0001 (DU diameter)
Ambrisentan	[146]	10 mg daily	SSc-vascular	RCT	12 weeks	15/5	>0.05 (blood flow), 0.005 (HAQ)

http://dx.doi.org/10.5772/66642

Study treatment	Ref.	Treatment dosage	Disease aspect studied	Study type	Duration of study	Number drug/ control	*p*-value (measure)
Macitentan	[115]	3/10 mg daily	SSc-DU	RCT (x2)	16 weeks	192/97 176/89	>0.05 (DU formation)
Other agents							
Fasudil	[116]	40/80 mg	SSc-RP	RCT crossover	Various	17/0	>0.05 (blood flow recovery)
ORM-12741	[117]	30/100 mg	SSc-RP	RCT crossover	Various	12/0	>0.05 (blood flow recovery)

Ref. = study reference, *Number drug/control* = number of subjects in the treatment and control arms of the study, and *p-value (measure)* = statistical significance of the outcome measure defined in brackets.
TNFα, tumour necrosis factor alpha; *CYC,* cyclophosphamide; *SSc,* systemic sclerosis; *dcSSc,* diffuse cutaneous systemic sclerosis; *CTD,* connective tissue disorder; *SSc-ILD,* systemic sclerosis-associated interstitial lung disease; *SSc-m'skel,* systemic sclerosis-associated musculoskeletal manifestations; *SSc-skin,* systemic sclerosis-associated skin manifestations; *SSc-vascular,* systemic sclerosis-associated vascular manifestations; *SSc-DU,* systemic sclerosis-associated digital ulcers; *SSc-PAH,* systemic sclerosis-associated pulmonary arterial hypertension; *SSc-NDU,* systemic sclerosis-associated nondigital ulceration; *SSc-RP,* systemic sclerosis-associated Raynaud's phenomenon; *RCT,* randomised-controlled trial; *mRSS,* modified Rodman skin score; *PFTs,* pulmonary function tests; *FVC,* forced vital capacity; *HAQ,* health assessment questionnaire; *DAS28,* disease activity score at 28 joints; *DLco,* diffusing capacity of carbon monoxide; *PBP,* peripheral blood perfusion; *DU,* digital ulcer; *RP,* Raynaud's phenomenon; *6MWD* 6-min walking distance; *NYHA class,* New York Heart Association Functional Classification of Heart Failure; *FMD,* flow-mediated dilatation; *RV mass,* right ventricular mass; *PVR,* pulmonary vascular resistance; *N/A,* not applicable/ specified.

Table 1. Clinical studies of targeted therapies in systemic sclerosis published during the last 10 years.

2.1. Fibrosis

2.1.1. TGF-β pathway inhibitors

Central to the fibroblast-mediated overproduction of extracellular matrix and perturbed tissue repair in SSc are a number of pro-fibrotic growth factors, the most notable of which is transforming growth factor-β (TGF-β). The TGF-β pathway has been strongly implicated in the pathogenesis of systemic sclerosis in numerous *in vitro* and *in vivo* studies. One such example is the reduction in fibrosis seen in mouse models following the abrogation of TGF-β signalling [33, 34]. As such, the TGF-β pathway has been the focus of a number of studies in the search for targeted therapies for SSc, with several different approaches tested.

A logical approach is to target the growth factors themselves using neutralising antibodies. One of the first anti-TGF-β antibodies to be trialled in SSc was CAT-192, a recombinant human antibody against the TGF-β1 isoform. In Denton et al.'s pioneering study, CAT-192 was administered at different doses to a cohort of patients with early dcSSc using a randomised, double-blind, placebo-controlled study design [35]. Of the 45 patients enrolled into the study, 31 patients completed the trial. Four patients who received CAT-192 died during the study, although these deaths were thought to be a consequence of the underlying disease as opposed to a direct result of treatment with CAT-192. Skin sclerosis scores, as determined by the modified Rodman skin score (mRSS), did not demonstrate any significant treatment effect for CAT-192, with a global improvement in mRSS occurring independently of CAT-192 treatment. Similarly, no significant differences were noted in pulmonary function or functional status, as determined by the Scleroderma Health Assessment Questionnaire (HAQ). Furthermore, an excess of adverse events and severe adverse events was noted in the CAT-192 treatment group, although the majority were thought not to be related to treatment.

As noted by Denton et al., the lack of efficacy shown by CAT-192 could possibly be explained by its relatively weak affinity for only one isoform of TGF-β ligand. They suggest that abrogation of all active isoforms of the TGF-β ligand might induce a greater anti-fibrotic effect, as demonstrated in animal models [35]. Importantly, however, the desire to abrogate pro-fibrotic pathways must be balanced against the loss of their normal physiological functions, including potential tumour-suppressant roles [36].

Fresolimumab is a neutralising antibody targeting all three isoforms of TGF-β. Rice et al. conducted an open-label pilot study of fresolimumab in 15 patients with early dcSSc, employing two different dosing schedules [37]. mRSS values were shown to improve significantly by 3 weeks ($p = 0.0002$), with the changes remaining significant at 17 weeks ($p = 0.0024$). The clinical improvements in skin thickness paralleled a decrease in the expression of TGF-β-related biomarkers in skin biopsies following fresolimumab treatment. Interestingly, by 24 weeks, the subjects' skin scores had begun to deteriorate, along with re-expression of the TGF-β-mediated biomarkers, suggesting progression of the underlying skin disease. This led the authors to question whether a longer course of treatment, or repeated treatments, might help to sustain the treatment response. This must be balanced against adverse treatment effects, however. Anaemia was the most commonly reported adverse event in the study, with 67% of subjects experiencing a decrease in haemoglobin levels of >10% from baseline. Bleeding from sites including the gastrointestinal tract, gums, eyes and nose was also reported in a number of patients.

Another anti-fibrotic agent thought to act, at least in part, by suppressing TGF-β signalling is pirfenidone. Pirfenidone is also thought to possess anti-inflammatory properties, with action against TNFα demonstrated in several studies [38, 39]. This dual anti-fibrotic and anti-inflammatory action makes pirfenidone an attractive candidate for use in SSc. Indeed, pirfenidone has been extensively studied in idiopathic pulmonary fibrosis, with several large phase III studies demonstrating improvements in progression-free survival [40, 41].

Khanna et al. recently studied pirfenidone in a 16-week, open-label study of 63 patients with SSc-associated interstitial lung disease (SSc-ILD) [42]. The primary aim of the study was to test pirfenidone's safety and tolerability in such patients. The vast majority of subjects did indeed experience adverse events during the course of the study, although most were mild or moderate in severity, with a similar adverse event profile to previous studies of pirfenidone in idiopathic pulmonary fibrosis. Median changes (from baseline) in the percentage of predicted forced vital capacity (FVC) and diffusing capacity of carbon monoxide (DLco) were non-significant, at -0.5% and +1.5%, respectively. Clinically insignificant changes in skin scores were also noted. Of note, the authors state clearly that this study was inadequately powered to assess efficacy.

Further studies are required before conclusions can be drawn on pirfenidone's efficacy in SSc. A case series of five patients with SSc-ILD treated with pirfenidone has provided hope of a potential benefit [43]. Vital capacity (as a percentage of predicted) was shown to improve by 12.2–28.9% in four patients following pirfenidone therapy, depending on the duration of follow-up. In the case of the fifth patient, vital capacity improved by a more modest 3.8% after pirfenidone therapy, albeit after only 3 months of follow-up. Furthermore, the authors noted that dyspnoea was attenuated in three patients, along with a reduction in ground-glass shadowing seen on the chest imaging of two patients. In another study of 12 patients, the potential benefits of topical pirfenidone in patients with localised scleroderma (morphoea) were demonstrated, with significant improvements seen in skin scores ($p = 0.002$) and histopathological markers ($p = 0.032$) at 6 months [44].

2.1.2. *Tyrosine kinase inhibitors*

Another approach is to target the downstream pathways induced by pro-fibrotic molecules such as TGF-β and platelet-derived growth factor (PDGF). The downstream pathways induced by these molecules require tyrosine kinase signalling [45]. Tyrosine kinase inhibitors are therefore strong candidates for use as anti-fibrotic agents in SSc. This is facilitated by the fact that several of these agents are already widely used in other conditions, such as in chronic myeloid leukaemia.

Pope et al. tested imatinib mesylate, an inhibitor of the BCR-ABL, c-kit and PDGF tyrosine kinase receptors, in a randomised, double-blind, placebo-controlled study of patients with active dcSSc over a 6-month period [45]. Outcomes measured included changes in skin scores, global assessments of patients' well-being and safety outcomes. Despite a plan to enrol 20 patients into the study, enrolment was cut short after 10 patients in view of the high observed number of adverse events. Side effects noted included diarrhoea, nausea, oedema and alopecia, with two patients requiring hospital admission. The tolerability remained poor despite a dose reduction from 200 mg twice daily to 200 mg once daily. Of the efficacy outcome measures assessed, no significant treatment effect was observed in skin scores or global assessment measures, although conclusions were limited by the small number of subjects and short study duration.

Focusing on SSC-associated lung fibrosis, Khanna et al. performed a 1-year, open-label study of imatinib in 20 SSc patients with active ILD [46]. Doses of up to 600 mg per day were used, with a mean dosage of 445 mg per day. In keeping with the outcome of Pope et al.'s study, 25% of subjects discontinued this study as a result of adverse events, with a similar profile of side effects noted. A modest, non-significant improvement in FVC was observed in patients receiving imatinib, coupled with a significant improvement in skin scores ($p < 0.001$). Further corroborating the results of this study, Spiera et al. demonstrated a significant improvement in skin scores ($p < 0.001$) and FVC ($p = 0.008$) in their open-label, 1-year study of imatinib 400 mg daily in 30 patients with dcSSc [47]. The improvements in skin scores seen in this study paralleled significant decreases in skin thickness as evident on skin biopsy ($p < 0.01$). Again, a large number of adverse events were noted in this study, with 171 adverse events thought to be at least possibly related to imatinib. A 24-month open-label extension of this study demonstrated ongoing improvement in skin scores ($p = 0.002$) [48].

More recently, a phase II open-label study recruited 30 patients with active SSc-ILD, unresponsive to cyclophosphamide, and administered a lower dose of 200 mg daily of imatinib for 6 months [49]. Following an additional 6 months of follow-up, a range of respiratory outcome measures were assessed (with a 'good response' defined as an increase in FVC and/or DLco of >15%, combined with a PaO2 of >90% of the initial value and stable/improved lung imaging). Of the 26 subjects who completed the study, 4 subjects demonstrated a good response, 15 subjects had stable lung disease and 7 subjects had a worsening of their lung disease. Although fewer patients reached the criteria of 'good response' than their goal of 30%, the authors pointed out that their cohort of patients had advanced lung disease, unresponsive to conventional cyclophosphamide therapy. They suggested that a cohort of patients with earlier disease might experience greater benefit from imatinib therapy. Importantly, the lower dose of imatinib employed in this study was relatively well tolerated, with adverse events present in less than 20% of patients.

A second-generation tyrosine kinase inhibitor, nilotinib, was recently tested in an open-label pilot study of 10 patients with early dcSSc [50]. Nilotinib has been shown to have a favourable side-effect profile relative to imatinib when used in chronic myeloid leukaemia patients [50]. In the seven patients who completed the study, significant reductions were seen in skin scores after 6 months and 12 months of follow-up (p = 0.02 and 0.01, respectively). Significant improvements were also evident in the physician global assessment ($p = 0.0013$ at 12 months), although no significant differences were evident in measures of lung function. Seventy-one adverse events, including two serious adverse events, were reported in the study, with asymptomatic elevations in liver function tests and QTc prolongation being common adverse events.

2.1.3. Other agents

Another study employed a different approach when searching for novel targeted therapies for SSc [51]. Noting its proposed role as an autoantigen in SSc, the authors attempted to induce immune tolerance to type I collagen by administering it orally to 168 patients with dcSSc in a randomised, double-blind, placebo-controlled trial. In the primary efficacy outcome of mRSS, no significant differences were evident between the treated and placebo cohorts at 15 months. During subgroup analysis, the authors noted a significant reduction in mRSS in treated patients with late-phase disease ($p = 0.0063$), with the treatment effect first becoming apparent approximately 8 months after commencing treatment. Multiple adverse events were noted, although this was common to both the treated and placebo arms of the study.

Although named after its pregnancy-related functions, interest in recombinant human relaxin as a potential therapy for SSc stems from its ability to inhibit fibroblast-mediated collagen production and enhance collagen breakdown. A phase II, randomised, controlled study of recombinant human relaxin in patients with stable dcSSc demonstrated significant improvements in skin scores at 24 weeks, with evidence of benefit arising as early as 4 weeks into the follow-up period [52]. Following on from this study, Khanna et al. [53] performed a large phase

III study of relaxin at two doses in patients with dcSSc. Reductions in skin scores were noted in all groups, including placebo, with no significant differences between the study arms. No significant differences were evident in functional outcome measures and FVC deteriorated in patients receiving relaxin ($p < 0.04$). Furthermore, of the 36 subjects who dropped out of the study prematurely, 14 were as a result of adverse events, most notably of the renal system.

2.2. Inflammation

2.2.1. TNFα inhibitors

Given the success of TNFα inhibitors in other autoimmune rheumatological conditions, several studies have examined their use in SSc. Prior studies had shown that TNFα counters extracellular matrix production by fibroblasts *in vitro*, leading to concerns that TNFα inhibitors might potentiate fibrosis in SSc [54, 55]. This contrasted the results of several animal studies, where TNFα abrogation resulted in reductions in fibrosis [54, 56, 57]. It has been proposed that the effect of TNFα inhibition in SSc might vary depending on the stage of the disease. During the early inflammation-predominant phases of SSc, TNFα inhibitor-mediated suppression of inflammation may lead to a reduction in subsequent fibrosis, as seen in animal studies. This is supported by the enhanced expression of TNFα in leucocytes from patients with early SSc [58]. During the later fibrosis-predominant stages of SSc, TNFα inhibitor-mediated suppression of inflammation is less likely to be of significance and may even be pro-fibrotic in nature, as suggested by *in vitro* studies [54, 59].

Lam et al. conducted a retrospective analysis of 18 patients with scleroderma-associated joint disease who had been treated with etanercept, a decoy receptor that binds to circulating TNFα [60]. Concurrent treatment with other disease-modifying agents or corticosteroids was permitted in their analysis. Eighty-three percent of patients demonstrated a positive response to etanercept therapy, as determined by the treating physician on follow-up review. Mean HAQ scores and skin scores showed non-significant trends towards improvement ($p = 0.13$ and 0.12, respectively). Pulmonary function readings deteriorated during the course of etanercept therapy, albeit to a small degree, in keeping with the gradual decline in lung function seen in patients who did not receive etanercept therapy.

Infliximab, a chimaeric monoclonal antibody against TNFα, has also been tested in an open-label study of 16 patients with dcSSc [61]. In addition to a number of clinical outcome measures, several histopathological and serum correlates of collagen synthesis were measured. No significant difference was noted in skin scores at the 26-week end point, although a non-significant trend towards a lower mRSS was evident at 22 weeks ($p = 0.10$). Significant reductions were evident in the degree of type I collagen synthesis by dermal fibroblasts at 26 weeks ($p = 0.02$) and in the serum levels of aminoterminal propeptide of type III collagen ($p = 0.03$). Of the 127 adverse events that occurred during the course of the study, 19 adverse events were thought to be attributable to infliximab, with half of the patients prematurely discontinuing the therapy.

Following on from these studies, a multi-centre, retrospective analysis of TNFα inhibitor use in SSc was performed by the EULAR Scleroderma Trials and Research (EUSTAR) group [54].

Sixty-five patients who had received an anti-TNFα agent during the course of their treatment (most commonly infliximab and etanercept) were identified. Of the 65 patients analysed, 48 had shown evidence of improvement, with the majority of benefit seen in patients with joint-related symptoms. Improvements in fibrosis were less convincing, with six patients experiencing an improvement in fibrosis and seven patients experiencing a worsening of fibrosis. Using the Delphi technique to reach an expert consensus, 50% of centres ultimately recommended against using TNFα inhibitors in SSc other than in the setting of clinical trials, 9% of centres advised against their use entirely, and 38% of centres advocated consideration of TNFα inhibitors in SSc-associated joint disease.

2.2.2. Selective co-stimulation modulators

Abatacept is a fusion protein comprising the extracellular domain of human cytotoxic T-lymphocyte-associated antigen-4 (CTLA-4) and the modified Fc portion of human immunoglobulin G1 [62]. It is licensed as a treatment for moderate-to-severe rheumatoid arthritis that has failed to respond to conventional immunosuppressant therapy, and has been shown to have comparable efficacy to TNFα inhibitors [11, 63–65]. By binding to CD80/CD86 on the surface of antigen-presenting cells, abatacept inhibits the co-stimulatory interactions required for the activation of T-cells. T-cells have been strongly implicated in the pathogenesis of SSc and, as such, a number of studies have investigated the role of abatacept as a treatment for SSc [66, 67].

In a double-blind, placebo-controlled study, seven patients were randomised to receive abatacept and compared to three control patients [67]. Although limited by the small number of subjects, a trend towards improvement in absolute skin scores was noted with abatacept therapy at the 24-week end point ($p = 0.0625$). This improvement became statistically significant when the differences in disease duration between the two cohorts were accounted for ($p = 0.0114$). Patients receiving abatacept therapy also noted greater improvements in HAQ and visual analogue scores. Abatacept therapy was well tolerated, with no serious adverse events noted during the course of the study.

The EUSTAR group's observational study of two separate biological therapies—abatacept and tocilizumab (see below)—provides evidence to support abatacept's use in a cohort of patients with SSc-associated refractory arthritis [68]. Of the patients with joint disease receiving abatacept therapy, 6/11 reached the EULAR-specified criteria for a good response in their 28-joint count Disease Activity Score at 11 months. More impressive still was the 10/15 patients who achieved a good response in their joint scores following tocilizumab therapy after 5 months of follow-up. No benefit was seen in myopathic patients receiving abatacept therapy or in skin or lung fibrosis with either abatacept or tocilizumab therapy.

2.2.3. IL-2α inhibitors

Basiliximab, a chimaeric monoclonal antibody against CD25, disrupts T-cell action via a different mechanism to abatacept. The CD25 antigen corresponds to the alpha chain of the interleukin-2 (IL-2α) receptor, a transmembrane protein expressed on the surface of activated

T-cells [69]. By competing with IL-2 for access to its receptor, basiliximab disrupts the downstream effects of activated T-cells. Basiliximab has been utilised successfully as part of immunosuppressive regimens to prevent the acute rejection of transplanted organs [70]. The promising results of a phase II study of basiliximab in patients with skin fibrosis resulting from acute graft-versus-host disease also support its potential as a therapy for SSc [71].

Basiliximab was tested in an open-label, prospective study of 10 patients with rapidly progressive SSc [72]. As well as being relatively well tolerated, basiliximab therapy resulted in a significant improvement in skin scores by week 68 of follow-up ($p = 0.015$). A trend towards an improvement in mean FVC was also noted by week 44 ($p = 0.078$). Given the small size and open-label nature of this study, further trials are necessary before definitive comments can be made about basiliximab's efficacy in SSc. However, the results of this pilot study support the beneficial response seen in a case study of a patient with recalcitrant SSc, who responded favourably to basiliximab, in conjunction with cyclophosphamide [73].

2.2.4. IL-6 inhibitors

Tocilizumab is a humanised monoclonal antibody targeting the interleukin-6 (IL-6) receptor. As with abatacept and TNFα inhibitors, tocilizumab is an effective treatment for moderate-to-severe rheumatoid arthritis which has failed to respond adequately to conventional disease-modifying agents. In addition to its pro-inflammatory effects, IL-6 has been shown to be pro-fibrotic, as well as an endothelial cell activator [74, 75]. IL-6 levels are elevated in the serum of patients with dcSSc and predict poorer long-term clinical outcomes [75, 76].

Following on from the observational study of tocilizumab and abatacept in patients with SSc-associated joint disease (mentioned above), a case series published by Fernandes das Neves et al. demonstrated evidence of clinical improvement in three treatment-refractory SSc patients treated with tocilizumab [68, 77]. More recently, the safety and efficacy of tocilizumab in SSc was studied in a phase II, double-blind, randomised, placebo-controlled trial of 87 patients with a disease duration of less than 5 years [78]. A trend towards improvement was evident in the primary outcome (mean change in mRSS); however, this did not reach statistical significance at 48 weeks ($p = 0.0579$). No significant difference was evident in clinical symptoms or in global disease severity scores. However, significantly fewer patients in the tocilizumab cohort experienced a decline in FVC at 48 weeks ($p = 0.0373$). A relatively large number of patients in both cohorts experienced severe adverse events (33% treatment vs. 34% placebo), with a greater number of serious infections noted in the tocilizumab cohort and one death as a result of tocilizumab therapy. Further information about tocilizumab's efficacy and safety in SSc will be provided by the ongoing phase III study [79].

2.2.5. B-cell depletion

Rituximab is a chimaeric monoclonal antibody that targets the CD20 antigen, resulting in the depletion of peripheral B-cells. It has been shown to be highly effective in the treatment of rheumatoid arthritis, where it is often used as a rescue therapy for patients with refractory disease. Rituximab's clinical efficacy has to be weighed against the potential for serious side effects, which include infusion reactions, predisposition to infection and hypogammaglobulinaemia, and the serious but infrequent complication of progressive multifocal leukoencephalopathy.

A body of evidence supporting the role of B-cells in the pathogenesis of SSc has spurred interest in rituximab as a therapy for SSc. Indeed, B-cell depletion has been shown to suppress skin fibrosis and autoantibody production in mouse models of SSc, when utilised in early stages of the disease [80, 81]. An early, open-label, pilot study of rituximab in 15 patients with dcSSc produced disappointing results, however [82]. Although relatively safe and well tolerated, rituximab therapy failed to produce a significant improvement in skin scores after 6 and 12 months of follow-up ($p = 0.82$ and 0.83, respectively). This was despite demonstrable depletion of B-cells in the periphery and dermis. This pilot study has been followed by a number of studies which support the role of rituximab therapy in SSc [83–90].

In a 1-year prospective study by Daoussis et al., eight patients with SSc were randomised to receive two cycles of rituximab therapy, in addition to standard treatment, and compared to six patients who received standard treatment alone [87]. Relative to baseline, FVC improved significantly with rituximab therapy at the 1-year end point, with a median improvement of 10% ($p = 0.0018$). This was significantly improved relative to controls, where a median decline in FVC of 5% was evident ($p = 0.002$). Significant improvements were also evident in DLco and skin scores in the rituximab cohort ($p = 0.017$ and $p < 0.001$, respectively). An open-label extension of this study, whereby a further two cycles of rituximab therapy were administered, demonstrated ongoing improvements in FVC, DLco and skin scores at 2 years [88].

A 2-year, open-label, prospective study by Smith et al. [89] provided further evidence of rituximab's efficacy in SSc. Following two cycles of rituximab in eight patients with early dcSSc, statistically significant reductions in skin scores, disease activity scores and biomarkers of collagen deposition were evident by the 24-month end point ($p < 0.0001$, $p < 0.0001$ and $p = 0.009$, respectively). The EUSTAR group employed a retrospective case-control analysis to collate evidence on rituximab use in SSc across a number of centres [81]. Sixty-three patients were identified who had received rituximab during the course of their treatment. Several outcome measures were compared retrospectively to patients with SSc who had not received rituximab therapy. In patients treated with rituximab, mean skin scores were found to be significantly lower than baseline after a period of follow-up ($p = 0.0001$). In the subset of patients with severe dcSSc receiving rituximab, reductions in skin scores were significantly greater than matched controls ($p = 0.03$). Furthermore, patients with SSc-associated ILD experienced a stabilisation in their FVC following rituximab therapy, relative to matched controls ($p = 0.02$).

More recently, an open-label, prospective study of 30 SSc patients from three centres added further weight to the evidence base supporting rituximab's use in SSc [90]. Patients received four cycles of rituximab therapy over 18 months, followed by consideration for further cycles by their treating physician. After 1 and 2 years of follow-up, FVC had significantly improved relative to baseline ($p < 0.001$ and $p = 0.018$, respectively), with the same being true of DLco at 2 years ($P = 0.012$). By 5 years, FVC was shown to have stabilised ($p = 0.05$). Skin scores also improved significantly at all time points ($P < 0.001$). Again, rituximab was reported as being relatively well tolerated in this study.

http://dx.doi.org/10.5772/66642

Using a different approach, Schiopu et al. utilised a humanised anti-CD19 monoclonal antibody (MEDI-551) to deplete B-cells [91]. As noted by the authors, the CD19 antigen is expressed on a wider range of B-cell subsets than the CD20 antigen. In their study, 24 subjects were randomised to receive a single dose of MEDI-551 and compared to four subjects who received placebo therapy. The primary aim of the study was to test MEDI-551's safety and tolerability in SSc subjects. An excess of adverse events was indeed noted in the treatment cohort (95.8% of subjects) relative to the placebo cohort (75% of subjects), with the majority being mild or moderate events. Of the serious adverse events, two were thought possibly to have been a consequence of MEDI-551 treatment. Given that a number of studies of rituximab demonstrate the probable benefits of more prolonged B-cell depletion in SSc, this 85-day study of MEDI-551 was limited in its ability to discern clinical efficacy. A trend towards improvement in skin scores with MEDI-551 treatment was noted relative to placebo, although no clear evidence of benefit was seen in pulmonary function tests. Further studies are needed to determine its efficacy more conclusively.

2.2.6. Type I IFN receptor antagonists

Using another targeted approach to developing novel therapies for SSc, Goldberg et al. tested MEDI-546, a monoclonal antibody against the type I interferon (IFN) receptor, in patients with SSc [92]. Case reports have documented incident systemic sclerosis arising in patients who had previously received IFNα therapy for chronic viral hepatitis [93, 94]. An activated type I IFN profile and gene signature are present in patients with SSc and administration of MEDI-546 not only reduces serum levels of several IFN-induced proteins but also suppresses levels of markers of extracellular matrix turnover and TGF-β signalling [95, 96].

In a study designed to test MEDI-546's safety and tolerability in SSc, rather than its efficacy, Goldberg et al. administered the treatment to 34 subjects and recorded a range of safety, pharmacokinetic and immunogenicity outcomes after 12 weeks of follow-up [92]. Of the 148 adverse events, four were recorded as serious adverse events, one of which was a new diagnosis of chronic myelogenous leukaemia occurring after 10 months. Phase II, placebo-controlled studies are necessary before MEDI-546's efficacy in SSc can be commented on. Indeed, phase II studies of MEDI-546 are already ongoing in systemic lupus erythematosus (SLE).

2.3. Vascular

2.3.1. Endothelin receptor antagonists

The vasculopathy seen in SSc is characterised by endothelial cell damage and dysfunction and fibrotic obliteration of the vasculature, with consequent ischaemia-reperfusion injury [97]. This, in turn, stimulates the production of the potent vasoconstrictor, endothelin, which has been strongly implicated as a mediator of vascular injury in SSc. The vascular manifestations that result from these pathogenic processes include Raynaud's phenomenon (RP) and digital ulceration, pulmonary arterial hypertension (PAH) and renal crises.

One of few licensed targeted therapies for SSc is bosentan. Bosentan disrupts the endothelin-signalling axis by antagonising both of its receptors, endothelin-A and endothelin-B. Bosentan has been shown in a large number of studies to be an effective treatment for PAH, including SSc-associated PAH (SSc-PAH). Its use leads to improvements in symptoms, exercise capacity and a range of haemodynamic values [98, 99]. Several studies have also investigated bosentan's efficacy for the other vascular manifestations of SSc, most notably RP and digital ulceration, details of which are given below.

The RAPIDS-2 study was a large randomised, placebo-controlled trial designed to evaluate bosentan's efficacy in the treatment of SSc-associated digital ulcers. One hundred and eighty-eight patients with SSc and active digital ulcers were recruited from a number of centres, of which 98 were administered bosentan over the course of 20 weeks [100]. At the 24-week end point, a 30% reduction in the number of new digital ulcers was evident in the cohort receiving bosentan ($p = 0.04$). No significant difference was evident in ulcer healing time, however. The beneficial effects of bosentan on reducing digital ulcer formation are supported by two further studies—a retrospective analysis of 67 patients and a 3-year prospective, open-label study [101, 102]. Although generally well tolerated, all three studies demonstrated bosentan's well-documented side effect of inducing liver dysfunction. This is reversible in the vast majority of cases, although close monitoring of liver function during therapy is essential. This is highlighted by the results of a small study of bosentan in patients with SSc-associated digital ulcers, during which 50% of patients had to discontinue bosentan due to severe liver dysfunction [103].

It has been proposed that the differential effects of bosentan on digital ulcer formation and healing might stem from various pro- and anti-vasoconstrictive effects of the medication [104]. Ambrisentan also targets the endothelin axis but does so by selectively antagonising the endothelin-A receptor, as opposed to the dual-receptor blockade mediated by bosentan. The effects of ambrisentan on SSc-associated digital ulcer number and healing were analysed in a prospective, open-label study of 20 patients [104]. A significant decrease in the number of digital ulcers per patient was noted at 24 weeks relative to baseline ($p < 0.004$). The maximum diameter of patients' digital ulcers was also noted to decrease ($p < 0.0001$), and 88% of patients who completed the study had full resolution of all their baseline digital ulcers. Importantly, no study subjects developed deranged liver function tests during the course of this study.

The efficacy of ambrisentan in patients with SSc-PAH has also been tested in a prospective, open-label study [105]. Twenty-four patients with treatment-naïve SSc-PAH were administered dual therapy with ambrisentan and tadalafil, a phosphodiesterase type-5 inhibitor, for 36 weeks. Following this course of treatment, significant reductions were noted in pulmonary vascular resistance ($p < 0.0001$) and right ventricular mass ($p < 0.05$), as well as improvements in 6-min walk distances ($p = 0.001$) and other haemodynamic and structural outcome measures. These results are supported by those of another study, in which 12 patients with SSc-associated exercise-induced PAH experienced significant improvements in exercise-pulmonary vascular resistance and 6-min walk distances following 24 weeks of treatment with ambrisentan ($p =$ 0.004 and 0.003, respectively) [106].

Ambrisentan has also been shown to reduce the incidence of SSc-associated Raynaud's phenomenon (SSc-RP) attacks, albeit it in a study of only six patients ($p = 0.01$) [107]. Bosentan's effect on SSc-RP has been more extensively studied, with mixed results. In a retrospective analysis of 14 patients, bosentan use was associated with a significant decrease in the number and duration of RP attacks ($p < 0.05$) [97]. An open-label prospective study of 15 patients with lcSSc-associated RP also demonstrated a significant reduction in the duration, frequency and intensity of RP attacks with bosentan use ($p < 0.05$) [108]. These findings contrast the results of a randomised, placebo-controlled study involving 16 subjects with SSc-RP (without pre-existing digital ulcers). Relative to placebo, no improvements in the duration, intensity or frequency of RP attacks were seen with bosentan use, despite improvements in functional scores.

In addition to endothelin's prominent role as a mediator of vascular injury in SSc, it has also been implicated in promoting fibrosis. *In vitro,* endothelin stimulates production and deposition of extracellular matrix by fibroblasts, as well as facilitating the pro-fibrotic properties of TGF-β [97, 109, 110]. Endothelin levels are also elevated in the serum and bronchoalveolar lavage fluid of patients with SSc-ILD [111]. In light of endothelin's reported pro-fibrotic roles, the effects of bosentan on SSc-associated skin and lung fibrosis have been tested in a number of studies.

In a prospective, placebo-controlled study of patients with SSc-ILD, 77 patients were randomised to receive bosentan and their 6-min walk distances and oxygen saturations compared to 86 controls [112]. At 12 months, no significant difference was evident in walking distances between the study cohorts ($p = 0.404$), with the same being true of pulmonary function test results. Furuya et al. also examined bosentan's use in SSc-ILD in a 24-month open-label trial of 9 patients who were deemed ineligible for cyclophosphamide therapy [113]. Of the 7 patients who completed the study, a trend towards improvement in FVC, DLco and total lung capacity was noted. This contrasted the findings on high-resolution computed tomography (CT) thorax scans, which showed a gradual progression of the underlying fibrosis. Moreover, no benefit on cumulative survival was evident when the subjects were compared to historical controls.

Bosentan's effect on skin fibrosis was evaluated in a retrospective, open-label study of 14 patients who were receiving bosentan for SSc-PAH [97]. As well as noting reductions in the duration and number of RP attacks, significant reductions in skin scores were present in the study cohort after 24 weeks of follow-up ($p < 0.01$). The retrospective nature of this study and the lack of control subjects both necessitate a degree of caution when interpreting these results, particularly as spontaneous regression of skin disease is not uncommonly seen in SSc patients. Indeed, Seibold et al.'s placebo-controlled study of bosentan in SSc-ILD (described above) failed to show any significant treatment effect on skin thickness scores. This contrasts the results of another, albeit much smaller, prospective study which did highlight a significant improvement in mRSS with bosentan therapy ($p < 0.001$) [114]. Again, the lack of control subjects in this study makes it difficult to separate bosentan's effects on skin scores from the improvements sometimes seen in the natural progression of SSc.

Another endothelin-receptor antagonist to have been studied in SSc is macitentan. Like bosentan, macitentan acts to antagonise both of the endothelin receptors, albeit with a much greater affinity for the endothelin-A receptor. Macitentan's effects on SSc-associated digital ulcers were recently studied in two phase III placebo-controlled trials with a total of 554 study subjects [115]. After 16 weeks of follow-up, no significant treatment effect was evident in the primary end point of cumulative number of new digital ulcers. The same was true of the secondary end points of digital ulcer healing, total ulcer burden and hand function.

2.3.2. *Other agents*

Two other targeted vascular therapies worthy of mention are fasudil and ORM-12741, both of which have primary targets outside of the endothelin axis. Fasudil is a RhoA/Rho kinase inhibitor that abrogates the α2C-adrenoceptor-mediated response to cold exposure, whereas ORM-12741 acts as a direct α2C-adrenoceptor antagonist. When studied in patients with SSc-associated RP, neither agent enhanced recovery in blood flow nor skin temperature following cold challenges [116, 117]. Although unsuccessful in their trials to date, fasudil and ORM-12741 provide us with further examples of how research into the pathogenesis of SSc can be translated into novel candidates for drug therapies.

3. Conclusion

In this chapter, we have reviewed a wide range of targeted therapies for SSc. Our systematic literature search identified 69 clinical studies of targeted therapies with diverse modes of action. This reflects the concerted efforts of clinicians and researchers trying to identify novel therapies for this disabling condition.

Progress has already been made in improving the outlook for certain groups of patients with SSc. Autologous haematopoietic stem cell transplantation, for example, has been shown to benefit patients with early, aggressive dcSSc. Unfortunately, this benefit comes at the expense of significant treatment-related morbidity and mortality, thereby limiting the utility of this treatment for the majority of patients with SSc.

The discovery of efficacious targeted therapies has the potential to transform the outlook for patients with SSc, just as TNFα inhibitors have done in rheumatoid arthritis, psoriatic arthritis and ankylosing spondylitis. In this regard, most progress has been made in developing targeted therapies for the vascular manifestations of SSc. The endothelin-receptor antagonists bosentan and ambrisentan have been tested in more than 30 clinical studies involving patients with SSc. As detailed above, many of these studies have demonstrated statistically significant treatment effects on vascular manifestations such as PAH and digital ulcer formation. A phase II study of zibotentan, a selective endothelin-receptor A antagonist, is also currently underway for patients with SSc-associated renal dysfunction [118].

Improvements in our understanding of another of the central pillars of SSc pathogenesis – fibrosis – have also been made. The studies of the anti-TGF-β antibodies, CAT-192 and fresolimumab, are excellent examples of how an understanding of the pathogenic processes underlying SSc can be translated into targeted therapies. The improvements seen in skin fibrosis scores following treatment with fresolimumab provide us with an exciting glimpse of the potential benefits of targeted anti-fibrotic therapies. This excitement is partly tempered by

http://dx.doi.org/10.5772/66642

the large number of adverse events seen in this study; a clear reminder of the potential pitfalls of disturbing physiological functions, such as fibrosis and healing.

Of the targeted anti-inflammatory therapies, a great deal of optimism can be derived from the studies of rituximab, a B-cell-depleting antibody with efficacy in a wide range of clinical conditions. Of the 10 studies identified that assessed rituximab in SSc, 9 demonstrated statistically significant treatment effects. Moreover, 6 of these studies revealed treatment benefits in measures of both skin and lung fibrosis. Rituximab also provides us with an example of how an existing targeted therapy can be adopted for use in SSc. Analysis of safety and efficacy data from studies in other conditions can help tailor the design of studies of rituximab in SSc and expedite the transition process.

As demonstrated in **Table 1**, a large number of the trials involving targeted therapies in SSc have been small, open-label studies. Their limited size and, in many cases, lack of control subjects reduces the reliability of their outcome data. Large randomised, placebo-controlled studies are essential before definitive conclusions can be drawn about a particular treatment. Performing such studies in SSc is challenging given the rarity of the condition and the heterogeneity in its presentation and natural progression. Multi-centre collaboration can help to overcome these barriers by increasing the pool of subjects available for trials. Indeed, multi-centre randomised, controlled trials have already been performed for bosentan, macitentan, tocilizumab, MEDI-551, relaxin, oral type-I collagen, CAT-192 and imatinib mesylate. A number of large randomised, placebo-controlled trials are also ongoing for several of the therapies covered in this chapter. Examples include the ASSET trial—a phase II study of abatacept's efficacy in dcSSc—and the focuSSced trial—a phase III study of tocilizumab in SSc [79, 119].

A better understanding of the pathogenic processes underlying SSc will help to reduce the heterogeneity of study cohorts in trials of SSc. Stratification of patients into cohorts with specific biochemical or clinical characteristics will permit tailoring of treatments to those patients most likely to benefit. For example, an anti-cytokine therapy might be offered to those patients with a cytokine profile that suggests they are likely to benefit from such a therapy.

An improved understanding of the pathogenic processes underlying SSc will also increase the number of available drug targets. Trials are currently underway for a number of agents with novel mechanisms of action. The pan-peroxisome proliferator-activated receptor (PPAR) agonist, IVA337, is currently being investigated in a phase II randomised, controlled study of patients with dcSSc [120]. The anti-fibrotic properties of PPAR agonists are supported by the results of a recent study in a mouse model of dermal fibrosis, in which IVA337 administration produced reductions in extracellular matrix deposition and several biomarkers of inflammation and fibrosis [121]. Also promising is the ongoing phase III study of nintedanib in patients with SSc-ILD [122]. Nintedanib is a tyrosine kinase inhibitor that targets the receptors of vascular endothelial growth factor, fibroblast growth factor and PDGF. It has been shown to retard the progression of idiopathic pulmonary fibrosis in phase III studies and reduce fibrosis in multiple mouse models of SSc [123, 124]. Another candidate therapy worthy of mention is riociguat, a soluble guanylate cyclase stimulator that possesses both vasodilatory and anti-fibrotic properties. Riociguat has been shown to improve exercise capacity and several other haemodynamic and functional outcomes in patients with symptomatic PAH, and its effects on measures of skin and lung fibrosis are currently being assessed in a phase II study of patients with dcSSc [125].

Author details

Mark D. Russell* and Nidhi Sofat

*Address all correspondence to: mdrussell@doctors.org.uk

Institute of Infection and Immunity, St George's, University of London, United Kingdom

References

[1] Buchan G, Barrett K, Turner M, et al. Interleukin-1 and tumour necrosis factor mRNA expression in rheumatoid arthritis: Prolonged production of IL-1 alpha. Clinical and Experimental Immunology. 1988;73(3):449–55.

[2] Chu CQ, Field M, Feldmann M, et al. Localization of tumor necrosis factor alpha in synovial tissues and at the cartilage-pannus junction in patients with rheumatoid arthritis. Arthritis and Rheumatism. 1991;34(9):1125–32.

[3] Williams RO, Feldmann M, Maini RN. Anti-tumor necrosis factor ameliorates joint disease in murine collagen-induced arthritis. Proceedings of the National Academy of Sciences of the United States of America. 1992;89(20):9784–8.

[4] Elliott MJ, Maini RN, Feldmann M, et al. Treatment of rheumatoid arthritis with chimeric monoclonal antibodies to tumor necrosis factor alpha. Arthritis and Rheumatism. 1993;36(12):1681–90.

[5] Elliott MJ, Maini RN, Feldmann M, et al. Repeated therapy with monoclonal antibody to tumour necrosis factor alpha (cA2) in patients with rheumatoid arthritis. Lancet. 1994;344(8930):1125–7.

[6] Elliott MJ, Maini RN, Feldmann M, et al. Randomised double-blind comparison of chimeric monoclonal antibody to tumour necrosis factor alpha (cA2) versus placebo in rheumatoid arthritis. Lancet. 1994;344(8930):1105–10.

[7] NICE. Adalimumab, etanercept and infliximab for the treatment of rheumatoid arthritis [Internet]. 2007. Available at: http://www.nice.org.uk/TA130 (Accessed: 27 September 2016).

[8] NICE. Adalimumab, etanercept, infliximab, rituximab and abatacept for the treatment of rheumatoid arthritis after the failure of a TNF inhibitor [Internet]. 2010. Available from: http://www.nice.org.uk/TA195 (Accessed: 27 September 2016).

[9] Nam JL, Ramiro S, Gaujoux-Viala C, et al. Efficacy of biological disease-modifying antirheumatic drugs: a systematic literature review informing the 2013 update of the EULAR recommendations for the management of rheumatoid arthritis. Annals of the Rheumatic Diseases. 2014;73(3):516–28. doi: 10.1136/annrheumdis-2013-204577

[10] Williams RO, Paleolog E, Feldmann M. Cytokine inhibitors in rheumatoid arthritis and other autoimmune diseases. Current Opinion in Pharmacology. 2007;7(4):412–7. doi: 10.1016/j.coph.2007.06.001

[11] NICE. Abatacept for treating rheumatoid arthritis after the failure of conventional disease-modifying anti-rheumatic drugs [Internet]. 2013. Available at: http://www.nice.org.uk/TA280 (Accessed: 27 September 2016).

[12] NICE. Tocilizumab for the treatment of rheumatoid arthritis [Internet]. 2012. Available at: http://www.nice.org.uk/TA247 (Accessed: 27 September 2016).

[13] NICE. Rheumatoid arthritis in adults: Management [Internet]. 2009. Available at: http://www.nice.org.uk/CG79 (Accessed: 27 September 2016).

[14] NICE. Etanercept, infliximab and adalimumab for the treatment of psoriatic arthritis [Internet]. 2010. Available at: http://www.nice.org.uk/TA199 (Accessed: 27 September 2016).

[15] NICE. Adalimumab, etanercept and infliximab for ankylosing spondylitis [Internet]. 2008. Available at: http://www.nice.org.uk/TA143 (Accessed: 27 September 2016).

[16] NICE. Abatacept, adalimumab, etanercept and tocilizumab for treating juvenile idiopathic arthritis [Internet]. 2015. Available at: http://www.nice.org.uk/TA373 (Accessed: 27 September 2016).

[17] NICE. Infliximab and adalimumab for the treatment of Crohn's disease [Internet]. 2010. Available at: http://www.nice.org.uk/TA187 (Accessed: 27 September 2016).

[18] NICE. Ustekinumab for treating active psoriatic arthritis [Internet]. 2015. Available at: http://www.nice.org.uk/TA340 (Accessed: 27 September 2016).

[19] NICE. Secukinumab for treating moderate to severe plaque psoriasis [Internet]. 2015. Available at: http://www.nice.org.uk/TA350 (Accessed: 27 September 2016).

[20] McInnes IB, Mease PJ, Kirkham B, et al. Secukinumab, a human anti-interleukin-17A monoclonal antibody, in patients with psoriatic arthritis (FUTURE 2): A randomised, double-blind, placebo-controlled, phase 3 trial. Lancet. 2015;386(9999):1137–46. doi: 10.1016/S0140-6736(15)61134-5

[21] NICE. Belimumab for treating active autoantibody-positive systemic lupus erythematosus [Internet]. 2016. Available at: https://www.nice.org.uk/guidance/TA397 (Accessed: 72 September 2016).

[22] Denton CP, Black CM, Abraham DJ. Mechanisms and consequences of fibrosis in systemic sclerosis. Nature Clinical Practice Rheumatology. 2006;2(3):134–44. doi: 10.1038/ncprheum0115

[23] Kowal-Bielecka O, Landewé R, Avouac J, et al. EULAR recommendations for the treatment of systemic sclerosis: A report from the EULAR Scleroderma trials and research group (EUSTAR). Annals of the Rheumatic Diseases. 2009;68(5):620–8. doi: 10.1136/ard.2008.096677

[24] Denton CP, Hughes M, Gak N, et al. BSR and BHPR guideline for the treatment of systemic sclerosis. Rheumatology (Oxford). 2016;55(10):1906–10. doi: 10.1093/rheumatology/kew224

[25] Denton CP. Systemic sclerosis: from pathogenesis to targeted therapy. Clinical and Experimental Rheumatology. 2015;33(4 Suppl 92):S3–7.

[26] van Laar JM, Farge D, Sont JK, et al. Autologous hematopoietic stem cell transplantation vs intravenous pulse cyclophosphamide in diffuse cutaneous systemic sclerosis: a randomized clinical trial. JAMA. 2014;311(24):2490–8. doi: 10.1001/jama.2014.6368

[27] Burt RK, Shah SJ, Dill K, et al. Autologous non-myeloablative haemopoietic stem-cell transplantation compared with pulse cyclophosphamide once per month for systemic sclerosis (ASSIST): an open-label, randomised phase 2 trial. Lancet. 2011;378(9790):498–506. doi: 10.1016/S0140-6736(11)60982-3

[28] Poelman CL, Hummers LK, Wigley FM, et al. Intravenous immunoglobulin may be an effective therapy for refractory, active diffuse cutaneous systemic sclerosis. The Journal of Rheumatology. 2014;42(2):236–42. doi: 10.3899/jrheum.140833

[29] Takehara K, Ihn H, Sato S. A randomized, double-blind, placebo-controlled trial: intravenous immunoglobulin treatment in patients with diffuse cutaneous systemic sclerosis. Clinical and Experimental Rheumatology. 2013;31(2 Suppl 76):151–6.

[30] Raja J, Nihtyanova SI, Murray CD, et al. Sustained benefit from intravenous immunoglobulin therapy for gastrointestinal involvement in systemic sclerosis. Rheumatology (Oxford). 2016;55(1):115–9. doi: 10.1093/rheumatology/kev318

[31] Nacci F, Righi A, Conforti ML, et al. Intravenous immunoglobulins improve the function and ameliorate joint involvement in systemic sclerosis: a pilot study. Annals of the Rheumatic Diseases. 2007;66(7):977–9. doi: 10.1136/ard.2006.060111

[32] Denton CP, Ong VH. Targeted therapies for systemic sclerosis. Nature Reviews Rheumatology. 2013;9(8):451–64. doi: 10.1038/nrrheum.2013.46

[33] McCormick LL, Zhang Y, Tootell E, et al. Anti-TGF-beta treatment prevents skin and lung fibrosis in murine sclerodermatous graft-versus-host disease: a model for human scleroderma. Journal of Immunology. 1999;163(10):5693–9.

[34] Ruzek MC, Jha S, Ledbetter S, et al. A modified model of graft-versus-host-induced systemic sclerosis (scleroderma) exhibits all major aspects of the human disease. Arthritis and Rheumatism. 2004;50(4):1319–31. doi: 10.1002/art.20160

[35] Denton CP, Merkel PA, Furst DE, et al. Recombinant human anti-transforming growth factor beta1 antibody therapy in systemic sclerosis: a multicenter, randomized, placebo-controlled phase I/II trial of CAT-192. Arthritis and Rheumatism;56(1):323–33. doi: 10.1002/art.22289

[36] Elliott RL, Blobe GC. Role of transforming growth factor beta in human cancer. Journal of Clinical Oncology. 2005;23(9):2078–93. doi: 10.1200/JCO.2005.02.047

[37] Rice LM, Padilla CM, McLaughlin SR, et al. Fresolimumab treatment decreases biomarkers and improves clinical symptoms in systemic sclerosis patients. The Journal of Clinical Investigation. 2015;125(7):2795–807. doi: 10.1172/JCI77958

[38] Grattendick KJ, Nakashima JM, Feng L, et al. Effects of three anti-TNF-alpha drugs: etanercept, infliximab and pirfenidone on release of TNF-alpha in medium and TNF-alpha associated with the cell in vitro. International Immunopharmacology. 2008;8(5): 679–87. doi: 10.1016/j.intimp.2008.01.013

[39] Oku H, Nakazato H, Horikawa T, et al. Pirfenidone suppresses tumor necrosis factor-alpha, enhances interleukin-10 and protects mice from endotoxic shock. European Journal of Pharmacology. 2002;446:167–76.

[40] King TE Jr, Bradford WZ, Castro-Bernardini S, et al. A phase 3 trial of pirfenidone in patients with idiopathic pulmonary fibrosis. The New England Journal of Medicine. 2014;370(22):2083–92. doi: 10.1056/NEJMoa1402582

[41] Noble PW, Albera C, Bradford WZ, et al. Pirfenidone in patients with idiopathic pulmonary fibrosis (CAPACITY): two randomised trials. Lancet. 2011;377(9779):1760–9. doi: 10.1016/S0140-6736(11)60405-4

[42] Khanna D, Albera C, Fischer A, et al. An open-label, phase II study of the safety and tolerability of Pirfenidone in patients with scleroderma-associated interstitial lung disease: the LOTUSS trial. The Journal of Rheumatology. 2016;43(9):1672–9. doi: 10.3899/jrheum.151322

[43] Miura Y, Saito T, Fujita K, et al. Clinical experience with pirfenidone in five patients with scleroderma-related interstitial lung disease. Sarcoidosis, Vasculitis and Diffuse Lung Diseases. 2014;31(3):235–8.

[44] Rodríguez-Castellanos M, Tlacuilo-Parra A, Sánchez-Enríquez S, et al. Pirfenidone gel in patients with localized scleroderma: a phase II study. Arthritis Research & Therapy. 2014;16(6):510. doi: 10.1186/s13075-014-0510-4

[45] Pope J, McBain D, Petrlich L, et al. Imatinib in active diffuse cutaneous systemic sclerosis: results of a six-month, randomized, double-blind, placebo-controlled, proof-

of-concept pilot study at a single center. Arthritis and Rheumatism. 2011;63(11):3547–51. doi: 10.1002/art.30549

[46] Khanna D, Saggar R, Mayes MD, et al. A one-year, phase I/IIa, open-label pilot trial of imatinib mesylate in the treatment of systemic sclerosis-associated active interstitial lung disease. Arthritis and Rheumatism. 2011;63(11):3540–6. doi: 10.1002/art.30548

[47] Spiera RF, Gordon JK, Mersten JN, et al. Imatinib mesylate (Gleevec) in the treatment of diffuse cutaneous systemic sclerosis: results of a 1-year, phase IIa, single-arm, open-label clinical trial. Annals of the Rheumatic Diseases. 2011;70(6):1003–9. doi: 10.1136/ard.2010.143974

[48] Gordon J, Udeh U, Doobay K, et al. Imatinib mesylate (Gleevec™) in the treatment of diffuse cutaneous systemic sclerosis: results of a 24-month open label, extension phase, single-centre trial. Clinical and Experimental Rheumatology. 2014;32(6 Suppl 86):S189–93.

[49] Fraticelli P, Gabrielli B, Pomponio G, et al. Low-dose oral imatinib in the treatment of systemic sclerosis interstitial lung disease unresponsive to cyclophosphamide: a phase II pilot study. Arthritis Research & Therapy. 2014;16(4);R144. doi: 10.1186/ar4606

[50] Gordon JK, Martyanov V, Magro C, et al. Nilotinib (Tasigna™) in the treatment of early diffuse systemic sclerosis: an open-label, pilot clinical trial. Arthritis Research & Therapy. 2015;17:213. doi: 10.1186/s13075-015-0721-3

[51] Postlethwaite AE, Wong WK, Clements P, et al. A multicenter, randomized, double-blind, placebo-controlled trial of oral type I collagen treatment in patients with diffuse cutaneous systemic sclerosis: I. oral type I collagen does not improve skin in all patients, but may improve skin in late-phase disease. Arthritis and Rheumatism. 2008;58(6):1810–22. doi: 10.1002/art.23501

[52] Seibold JR, Korn JH, Simms R, et al. Recombinant human relaxin in the treatment of scleroderma. a randomized, double-blind, placebo-controlled trial. Annals of Internal Medicine. 2000:132(11):871–9.

[53] Khanna D, Clements PJ, Furst DE, et al. Recombinant human relaxin in the treatment of systemic sclerosis with diffuse cutaneous involvement: a randomized, double-blind, placebo-controlled trial. Arthritis and Rheumatism;60(4):1102–11. doi: 10.1002/art.24380

[54] Distler JH, Jordan S, Airo P, et al. Is there a role for TNFα antagonists in the treatment of SSc? EUSTAR expert consensus development using the Delphi technique. Clinical and Experimental Rheumatology. 2011;29(2 Suppl 65):S40–5.

[55] Mauviel A, Daireaux M, Rédini F, et al. Tumor necrosis factor inhibits collagen and fibronectin synthesis in human dermal fibroblasts. FEBS Letters. 1988;236(1):47–52.

[56] Liu JY, Brass DM, Hoyle GW, et al. TNF-alpha receptor knockout mice are protected from the fibroproliferative effects of inhaled asbestos fibers. The American Journal of Pathology. 1998;153(6):1839–47.

[57] Piguet PF, Vesin C. Treatment by human recombinant soluble TNF receptor of pulmonary fibrosis induced by bleomycin or silica in mice. The European Respiratory Journal. 1994;7(3):515–8.

[58] Young V, Ho M, Vosper H, et al. Elevated expression of the genes encoding TNF-alpha and thromboxane synthase in leucocytes from patients with systemic sclerosis. Rheumatology (Oxford). 2002;41(8):869–75.

[59] Distler JH, Schett G, Gay S, et al. The controversial role of tumor necrosis factor alpha in fibrotic diseases. Arthritis and Rheumatism. 2008;58(8):2228–35. doi: 10.1002/art.23645

[60] Lam GK, Hummers LK, Woods A, et al. Efficacy and safety of etanercept in the treatment of scleroderma-associated joint disease. The Journal of Rheumatology. 2007;34(7):1636–7.

[61] Denton CP, Engelhart M, Tvede N, et al. An open-label pilot study of infliximab therapy in diffuse cutaneous systemic sclerosis. Annals of the Rheumatic Diseases. 2008;68(9):1433–9. doi: 10.1136/ard.2008.096123

[62] DrugBank: Abatacept [Internet]. Available from: http://www.drugbank.ca/drugs/DB01281. (Accessed: 27 September 2016).

[63] NICE. Adalimumab, etanercept, infliximab, certolizumab pegol, golimumab, tocilizumab and abatacept for rheumatoid arthritis not previously treated with DMARDs or after conventional DMARDs only have failed; 2016. Available at: https://www.nice.org.uk/guidance/TA375 (Accessed: 27 September 2016).

[64] Schiff M, Weinblatt ME, Valente R, et al. Head-to-head comparison of subcutaneous abatacept versus adalimumab for rheumatoid arthritis: two-year efficacy and safety findings from AMPLE trial. Annals of the Rheumatic Diseases. 2014;73(1):86–94. doi: 10.1136/annrheumdis-2013-203843

[65] Schiff M, Keiserman M, Codding C, et al. Efficacy and safety of abatacept or infliximab vs placebo in ATTEST: a phase III, multi-centre, randomised, double-blind, placebo-controlled study in patients with rheumatoid arthritis and an inadequate response to methotrexate. Annals of the Rheumatic Diseases. 2007;67(8):1096–103. doi: 10.1136/ard.2007.080002

[66] Chakravarty EF, Fiorentino D, Bennett M, et al. A pilot study of abatacept for the treatment of patients with diffuse cutaneous systemic sclerosis. Arthritis & Rheumatism. 2011;63(Suppl 10):707.

[67] Chakravarty EF, Martyanov V, Fiorentino D, et al. Gene expression changes reflect clinical response in a placebo-controlled randomized trial of abatacept in patients with diffuse cutaneous systemic sclerosis. Arthritis Research & Therapy. 2015;17:159. doi: 10.1186/s13075-015-0669-3

[68] Elhai M, Meunier M, Matucci-Cerinic M, et al. Outcomes of patients with systemic sclerosis-associated polyarthritis and myopathy treated with tocilizumab or abatacept:

a EUSTAR observational study. Annals of the Rheumatic Diseases. 2012;72(7):1217–20. doi: 10.1136/annrheumdis-2012-202657

[69] Salis P, Caccamo C, Verzaro R, et al. The role of basiliximab in the evolving renal transplantation immunosuppression protocol. Biologics: Targets & Therapy. 2008;2(2): 175–88.

[70] Thistlethwaite JR Jr, Nashan B, Hall M, et al. Reduced acute rejection and superior 1-year renal allograft survival with basiliximab in patients with diabetes mellitus. The global Simulect study group. Transplantation. 2000;70(5):784–90.

[71] Schmidt-Hieber M, Fietz T, Knauf W, et al. Efficacy of the interleukin-2 receptor antagonist basiliximab in steroid-refractory acute graft-versus-host disease. British Journal of Haematology. 2005:130(4):568–74. doi: 10.1111/j.1365-2141.2005.05631.x

[72] Becker MO, Brückner C, Scherer HU, et al. The monoclonal anti-CD25 antibody basiliximab for the treatment of progressive systemic sclerosis: an open-label study. Annals of the Rheumatic Diseases. 2010;70(7):1340–1. doi: 10.1136/ard.2010.137935

[73] Scherer HU, Burmester GR, Riemekasten G. Targeting activated T cells: successful use of anti-CD25 monoclonal antibody basiliximab in a patient with systemic sclerosis. Annals of the Rheumatic Diseases. 2006;65(9):1245–7. doi: 10.1136/ard.2005.046938

[74] Barnes TC, Anderson ME, Moots RJ. The many faces of interleukin-6: the role of IL-6 in inflammation, vasculopathy, and fibrosis in systemic sclerosis. International Journal of Rheumatology. 2011;2011:721608. doi: 10.1155/2011/721608

[75] Khan K, Xu S, Nihtyanova S, et al. Clinical and pathological significance of interleukin 6 overexpression in systemic sclerosis. Annals of the Rheumatic Diseases. 2012;71(7): 1235–42. doi: 10.1136/annrheumdis-2011-200955

[76] De Lauretis A, Sestini P, Pantelidis P, et al. Serum interleukin 6 is predictive of early functional decline and mortality in interstitial lung disease associated with systemic sclerosis. The Journal of Rheumatology. 2013;40(4):435–46. doi: 10.3899/jrheum.120725

[77] Fernandes das Neves M, Oliveira S, Amaral MC, et al. Treatment of systemic sclerosis with tocilizumab. Rheumatology (Oxford). 2015;54(2):371–2. doi: 10.1093/rheumatology/keu435

[78] Khanna D, Denton CP, Jahreis A, et al. Safety and efficacy of subcutaneous tocilizumab in adults with systemic sclerosis (faSScinate): a phase 2, randomised, controlled trial. Lancet. 2016;387(10038):2630–40. doi: 10.1016/S0140-6736(16)00232-4

[79] A study of the efficacy and safety of Tocilizumab in participants with systemic sclerosis (SSc) [focuSSced] [Internet]. 2015. Available at: https://clinicaltrials.gov/ct2/show/NCT02453256 (Accessed: 27 September 2016).

[80] Hasegawa M, Hamaguchi Y, Yanaba K, et al. B-lymphocyte depletion reduces skin fibrosis and autoimmunity in the tight-skin mouse model for systemic sclerosis. The American Journal of Pathology. 2006;169(3):954–66. doi: 10.2353/ajpath.2006.060205

[81] Jordan S, Distler JH, Maurer B, et al. Effects and safety of rituximab in systemic sclerosis: an analysis from the European Scleroderma trial and research (EUSTAR) group. Annals of the Rheumatic Diseases. 2015:74(6):1188–94. doi: 10.1136/annrheumdis-2013-204522

[82] Lafyatis R, Kissin E, York M, et al. B cell depletion with rituximab in patients with diffuse cutaneous systemic sclerosis. Arthritis and Rheumatism. 2009;60(2):578–83. doi: 10.1002/art.24249

[83] Moazedi-Fuerst FC, Kielhauser SM, Brickmann K, et al. Rituximab for systemic sclerosis: arrest of pulmonary disease progression in five cases. Results of a lower dosage and shorter interval regimen. Scandinavian Journal of Rheumatology. 2014;43(3):257–8. doi: 10.3109/03009742.2013.869617

[84] Smith V, van Praet JT, Vandooren B, et al. Rituximab in diffuse cutaneous systemic sclerosis: an open-label clinical and histopathological study. Annals of the Rheumatic Diseases. 2008;69(1):193–7. doi: 10.1136/ard.2008.095463

[85] Bosello S, De Santis M, Lama G, et al. B cell depletion in diffuse progressive systemic sclerosis: safety, skin score modification and IL-6 modulation in an up to thirty-six months follow-up open-label trial. Arthritis Research & Therapy. 2010;12(2):R54. doi: 10.1186/ar2965

[86] Daoussis D, Liossis SN, Antonopoulos I, et al. THU0245 Rituximab has a beneficial effect on lung function and skin fibrosis in patients with systemic sclerosis. An open label study. Annals of the Rheumatic Diseases. 2013;71(Suppl 3):237–238. doi: 10.1136/annrheumdis-2012-eular.2210

[87] Daoussis D, Liossis SN, Tsamandas AC, et al. Experience with rituximab in scleroderma: results from a 1-year, proof-of-principle study. Rheumatology (Oxford). 2010;49(2): 271–80. doi: 10.1093/rheumatology/kep093

[88] Daoussis D, Liossis SN, Tsamandas A, et al. Effect of long-term treatment with rituximab on pulmonary function and skin fibrosis in patients with diffuse systemic sclerosis. Clinical and Experimental Rheumatology. 2012;30(2 Suppl 71):S17–22.

[89] Smith V, Piette Y, van Praet JT, et al. Two-year results of an open pilot study of a 2-treatment course with rituximab in patients with early systemic sclerosis with diffuse skin involvement. The Journal of Rheumatology. 2012;40(1):52–7. doi: 10.3899/jrheum.120778

[90] Melissaropoulos K, Daoussis D, Antonopoulos I, et al. SAT0450 Rituximab in systemic sclerosis. Results of an up to seven years, open label, multicenter study with a follow-up of 89 patient-years. Annals of the Rheumatic Diseases. 2015;74(Suppl 2):823. doi: 10.1136/annrheumdis-2015-eular.4618

[91] Schiopu E, Chatterjee S, Hsu V, et al. Safety and tolerability of an anti-CD19 monoclonal antibody, MEDI-551, in subjects with systemic sclerosis: a phase I, randomized,

placebo-controlled, escalating single-dose study. Arthritis Research & Therapy. 2016;18(1):131. doi: 10.1186/s13075-016-1021-2

[92] Goldberg A, Geppert T, Schiopu E, et al. Dose-escalation of human anti-interferon-α receptor monoclonal antibody MEDI-546 in subjects with systemic sclerosis: a phase 1, multicenter, open label study. Arthritis Research & Therapy. 2014;16(1):R57. doi: 10.1186/ar4492

[93] Solans R, Bosch J, Esteban I, et al. Systemic sclerosis developing in association with the use of interferon alpha therapy for chronic viral hepatitis. Clinical and Experimental Rheumatology. 2004;22(5):625–8.

[94] Tahara H, Kojima A, Hirokawa T, et al. Systemic sclerosis after interferon alphacon-1 therapy for hepatitis C. Internal Medicine (Tokyo, Japan). 2007;46(8):473–6.

[95] Eloranta ML, Franck-Larsson K, Lövgren T, et al. Type I interferon system activation and association with disease manifestations in systemic sclerosis. Annals of the Rheumatic Diseases. 2010;69(7):1396–402. doi: 10.1136/ard.2009.121400

[96] Guo X, Higgs BW, Bay-Jensen AC, et al. Suppression of T cell activation and collagen accumulation by an Anti-IFNAR1 mAb, Anifrolumab, in adult patients with systemic sclerosis. The Journal of Investigative Dermatology. 2015;135(10):2402–9. doi: 10.1038/jid.2015.188

[97] Giordano N, Puccetti L, Papakostas P, et al. Bosentan treatment for Raynauds phenomenon and skin fibrosis in patients with systemic sclerosis and pulmonary arterial hypertension: an open-label, observational, retrospective study. International Journal of Immunopathology and Pharmacology. 2010;23(4):1185–94.

[98] Liu C, Chen J, Gao Y, et al. Endothelin receptor antagonists for pulmonary arterial hypertension. The Cochrane Database of Systematic Reviews. 2013;(2):CD004434.

[99] Launay D, Sitbon O, Le Pavec J, et al. Long-term outcome of systemic sclerosis-associated pulmonary arterial hypertension treated with bosentan as first-line monotherapy followed or not by the addition of prostanoids or sildenafil. Rheumatology (Oxford). 2010;49(3):490–500. doi: 10.1093/rheumatology/kep398

[100] Matucci-Cerinic M, Denton CP, Furst DE, et al. Bosentan treatment of digital ulcers related to systemic sclerosis: results from the RAPIDS-2 randomised, double-blind, placebo-controlled trial. Annals of the Rheumatic Diseases. 2011;70(1):32–8. doi: 10.1136/ard.2010.130658

[101] Roman Ivorra JA, Simeon CP, Alegre Sancho JJ, et al. Bosentan in clinical practice for treating digital and other ischemic ulcers in Spanish patients with systemic sclerosis: IBER-DU cohort study. The Journal of Rheumatology. 2011;38(8):1631–5. doi: 10.3899/jrheum.101266

[102] Tsifetaki N, Botzoris V, Alamanos Y, et al. Bosentan for digital ulcers in patients with systemic sclerosis: a prospective 3-year followup study. The Journal of Rheumatology. 2009;36(7):1550–2. doi: 10.3899/jrheum.080992

[103] Nagai Y, Hasegawa M, Hattori T, et al. Bosentan for digital ulcers in patients with systemic sclerosis. The Journal of Dermatology. 2012;39(1):48–51. doi: 10.1111/j.1346-8138.2011.01299.x

[104] Chung L, Ball K, Yaqub A, et al. Effect of the endothelin type A-selective endothelin receptor antagonist ambrisentan on digital ulcers in patients with systemic sclerosis: results of a prospective pilot study. Journal of the American Academy of Dermatology; 71(2):400–1. doi: 10.1016/j.jaad.2014.04.028

[105] Hassoun PM, Zamanian RT, Damico R, et al. Ambrisentan and Tadalafil up-front combination therapy in scleroderma-associated pulmonary arterial hypertension. American Journal of Respiratory and Critical Care Medicine. 2015;192(9):1102–10. doi: 10.1164/rccm.201507-1398OC

[106] Saggar R, Khanna D, Shapiro S, et al. Exercise induced pulmonary hypertension in systemic sclerosis and treatment with Ambrisentan: A prospective single center, open label, pilot study. In: Proceedings of the American Thoracic Society International Conference (ATS 2011); 13–18 May 2011. doi: 10.1164/ajrccm-conference.2011.183.1_MeetingAbstracts.A5885

[107] Parisi S, Peroni CL, Laganà A, et al. Efficacy of ambrisentan in the treatment of digital ulcers in patients with systemic sclerosis: a preliminary study. Rheumatology (Oxford). 2013;52(6):1142–4. doi: 10.1093/rheumatology/ket019

[108] Hettema ME, Zhang D, Bootsma H, et al. Bosentan therapy for patients with severe Raynaud's phenomenon in systemic sclerosis. Annals of the Rheumatic Diseases. 2007;66(10):1398–9. doi: 10.1136/ard.2007.073684

[109] Shi-Wen X, Chen Y, Denton CP, et al. Endothelin-1 promotes myofibroblast induction through the ETA receptor via a rac/phosphoinositide 3-kinase/Akt-dependent pathway and is essential for the enhanced contractile phenotype of fibrotic fibroblasts. Molecular Biology of the Cell. 2004;15(6):2707–19. doi: 10.1091/mbc.E03-12-0902

[110] Shi-Wen X, Kennedy L, Renzoni EA, et al. Endothelin is a downstream mediator of profibrotic responses to transforming growth factor beta in human lung fibroblasts. Arthritis and Rheumatism. 2007;56(12):4189–94. doi: 10.1002/art.23134

[111] Reichenberger F, Schauer J, Kellner K, et al. Different expression of endothelin in the bronchoalveolar lavage in patients with pulmonary diseases. Lung. 2002;179(3):163–74. doi: 10.1007/s004080000058

[112] Seibold JR, Denton C, Furst DE, et al. Randomized, prospective, placebo-controlled trial of bosentan in interstitial lung disease secondary to systemic sclerosis. Arthritis and Rheumatism. 2010;62(7):2101–8. doi: 10.1002/art.27466

[113] Furuya Y, Kuwana M. Effect of Bosentan on systemic sclerosis-associated interstitial lung disease ineligible for cyclophosphamide therapy: a prospective open-label study. The Journal of Rheumatology. 2011;38(10):2186–92. doi: 10.3899/jrheum.110499

[114] Kuhn A, Haust M, Ruland V, et al. Effect of bosentan on skin fibrosis in patients with systemic sclerosis: a prospective, open-label, non-comparative trial. Rheumatology (Oxford). 2010;49(7):1336–45. doi: 10.1093/rheumatology/keq077

[115] Khanna D, Denton CP, Merkel PA, et al. Effect of Macitentan on the development of new ischemic digital ulcers in patients with systemic sclerosis: DUAL-1 and DUAL-2 Randomized clinical trials. JAMA. 2016;315(18):1975–88. doi: 10.1001/jama.2016.5258

[116] Fava A, Wung PK, Wigley FM, et al. Efficacy of Rho kinase inhibitor fasudil in secondary Raynaud's phenomenon. Arthritis Care & Research (Hoboken). 2012;64(6):925–9. doi: 10.1002/acr.21622

[117] Herrick AL, Murray AK, Ruck A, et al. A double-blind, randomized, placebo-controlled crossover trial of the α2C-adrenoceptor antagonist ORM-12741 for prevention of cold-induced vasospasm in patients with systemic sclerosis. Rheumatology (Oxford). 2014;53(5):948–52. doi: 10.1093/rheumatology/ket421

[118] Zibotentan better renal Scleroderma outcome study - full text view [Internet]. 2014. Available at: https://clinicaltrials.gov/show/NCT02047708 (Accessed: 27 September 2016).

[119] A study of Subcutaneous Abatacept to treat diffuse cutaneous systemic sclerosis [Internet]. 2014. Available at: https://clinicaltrials.gov/ct2/show/NCT02161406 (Accessed: 27 September 2016).

[120] Proof-of-concept trial of IVA337 in diffuse cutaneous systemic sclerosis [Internet]. 2015. Available at: https://clinicaltrials.gov/show/NCT02503644 (Accessed: 27 September 2016).

[121] Ruzehaji N, Frantz C, Ponsoye M, et al. Pan PPAR agonist IVA337 is effective in prevention and treatment of experimental skin fibrosis. Annals of the Rheumatic Diseases. 2016. doi: 10.1136/annrheumdis-2015-208029

[122] A trial to compare Nintedanib with placebo for patients with scleroderma related lung fibrosis [Internet]. 2015. Available at: https://clinicaltrials.gov/show/NCT02597933 (Accessed: 27 September 2016).

[123] Richeldi L, du Bois RM, Raghu G, et al. Efficacy and safety of nintedanib in idiopathic pulmonary fibrosis. The New England Journal of Medicine. 2014;370(22):2071–82. doi: 10.1056/NEJMoa1402584

[124] Huang J, Beyer C, Palumbo-Zerr K, et al. Nintedanib inhibits fibroblast activation and ameliorates fibrosis in preclinical models of systemic sclerosis. Annals of the Rheumatic Diseases. 2016;75(5):883–90. doi: 10.1136/annrheumdis-2014-207109

[125] Efficacy and safety of Riociguat in patients with systemic sclerosis [Internet]. 2014 Available at: https://clinicaltrials.gov/show/NCT02283762 (Accessed: 27 September 2016).

[126] Prey S, Ezzedine K, Doussau A, et al. Imatinib mesylate in scleroderma-associated diffuse skin fibrosis: a phase II multicentre randomized double-blinded controlled trial. The British Journal of Dermatology. 2012;167(5):1138–44. doi: 10.1111/j.1365-2133.2012.11186.x

[127] Guo L, Chen XX, Gu YY, et al. Low-dose imatinib in the treatment of severe systemic sclerosis: a case series of six Chinese patients and literature review. Clinical Rheumatology. 2012;31(9):1395–400. doi: 10.1007/s10067-012-2032-2

[128] Tamaki Z, Asano Y, Hatano M, et al. Efficacy of low-dose imatinib mesylate for cutaneous involvement in systemic sclerosis: a preliminary report of three cases. Modern rheumatology/the Japan Rheumatism Association. 2011;22(1):94–9. doi: 10.1007/s10165-011-0472-1

[129] Sabnani I, Zucker MJ, Rosenstein ED, et al. A novel therapeutic approach to the treatment of scleroderma-associated pulmonary complications: safety and efficacy of combination therapy with imatinib and cyclophosphamide. Rheumatology (Oxford). 2008;48(1):49–52. doi: 10.1093/rheumatology/ken369

[130] De Paoli FV, Nielsen BD, Rasmussen F, et al. Abatacept induces clinical improvement in patients with severe systemic sclerosis. Scandinavian Journal of Rheumatology. 2014;43(4):342–5. doi: 10.3109/03009742.2013.812238

[131] Cutolo M, Ruaro B, Pizzorni C, et al. Longterm treatment with endothelin receptor antagonist bosentan and iloprost improves fingertip blood perfusion in systemic sclerosis. The Journal of Rheumatology. 2014;41(5):881–6. doi: 10.3899/jrheum.131284

[132] Romaniello A, Viola G, Salsano F, et al. In systemic sclerosis patients, bosentan is safe and effective for digital ulcer prevention and it seems to attenuate the development of pulmonary arterial hypertension. Rheumatology (Oxford). 2013;53(3):570–1. doi: 10.1093/rheumatology/ket424

[133] Taniguchi T, Asano Y, Hatano M, et al. Effects of bosentan on nondigital ulcers in patients with systemic sclerosis. The British Journal of Dermatology. 2011;166(2):417–21. doi: 10.1111/j.1365-2133.2011.10581.x

[134] Rosato E, Molinaro I, Borghese F, et al. Bosentan improves skin perfusion of hands in patients with systemic sclerosis with pulmonary arterial hypertension. The Journal of Rheumatology. 2010;37(12):2531–9. doi: 10.3899/jrheum.100358

[135] Nguyen VA, Eisendle K, Gruber I, et al. Effect of the dual endothelin receptor antagonist bosentan on Raynaud's phenomenon secondary to systemic sclerosis: a double-blind prospective, randomized, placebo-controlled pilot study. Rheumatology (Oxford). 2009;49(3):583–7. doi: 10.1093/rheumatology/kep413

[136] Funauchi M, Kishimoto K, Shimazu H, et al. Effects of bosentan on the skin lesions: an observational study from a single center in Japan. Rheumatology International. 2008;29(7):769–75. doi: 10.1007/s00296-008-0789-z

[137] Denton CP, Pope JE, Peter HH, et al. Long-term effects of bosentan on quality of life, survival, safety and tolerability in pulmonary arterial hypertension related to connective tissue diseases. Annals of the Rheumatic Diseases. 2007;67(9):1222–8. doi: 10.1136/ard.2007.079921

[138] García de la Peña-Lefebvre P, Rodríguez Rubio S, Valero Expósito M, et al. Long-term experience of bosentan for treating ulcers and healed ulcers in systemic sclerosis patients. Rheumatology (Oxford). 2008;47(4):464–6. doi: 10.1093/rheumatology/ken001

[139] Sfikakis PP, Papamichael C, Stamatelopoulos KS, et al. Improvement of vascular endothelial function using the oral endothelin receptor antagonist bosentan in patients with systemic sclerosis. Arthritis and Rheumatism. 2007;56(6):1985–93. doi: 10.1002/art.22634

[140] Moore TL, Vail A, Herrick AL. Assessment of digital vascular structure and function in response to bosentan in patients with systemic sclerosis-related Raynaud's phenomenon. Rheumatology (Oxford). 2006;46(2):363–4. doi: 10.1093/rheumatology/kel383

[141] Selenko-Gebauer N, Duschek N, Minimair G, et al. Successful treatment of patients with severe secondary Raynaud's phenomenon with the endothelin receptor antagonist bosentan. Rheumatology (Oxford). 2006;45(Suppl 3):iii45–8. doi: 10.1093/rheumatology/kel290

[142] Ahmadi-Simab K, Hellmich B, Gross WL. Bosentan for severe pulmonary arterial hypertension related to systemic sclerosis with interstitial lung disease. European Journal of Clinical Investigation. 2006;36(Suppl 3):44–8. doi: 10.1111/j.1365-2362.2006.01695.x

[143] Meijs J, Voskuyl AE, Bloemsaat-Minekus JP, et al. Blood flow in the hands of a predefined homogeneous systemic sclerosis population: the presence of digital ulcers and the improvement with bosentan. Rheumatology (Oxford). 2015;54(2):262–9. doi: 10.1093/rheumatology/keu300

[144] Denton CP, Humbert M, Rubin L, et al. Bosentan treatment for pulmonary arterial hypertension related to connective tissue disease: a subgroup analysis of the pivotal clinical trials and their open-label extensions. Annals of the Rheumatic Diseases. 2006;65(10):1336–40. doi: 10.1136/ard.2005.048967

[145] Chung L, Ball K, Yaqub A, et al. Effect of the endothelin type a-selective endothelin receptor antagonist ambrisentan on digital ulcers in patients with systemic sclerosis: results of a prospective pilot study. Journal of the American Academy of Dermatology. 2014;71(2):400–1. doi: 10.1016/j.jaad.2014.04.028

[146] Bose N, Bena J, Chatterjee S. Evaluation of the effect of ambrisentan on digital microvascular flow in patients with systemic sclerosis using laser Doppler perfusion imaging: a 12-week randomized double-blind placebo controlled trial. Arthritis Research & Therapy. 2015;17:44. doi: 10.1186/s13075-015-0558-9

Chapter 7

Myasthenia Gravis: Clinical and Immunological Aspects

Kokil Tandon

Additional information is available at the end of the chapter

http://dx.doi.org/10.5772/67684

Abstract

Autoimmune diseases such as myasthenia gravis (MG) result from an altered balance between the processes of activation and regulation of immune response. MG is the most common autoimmune disorder characterized by failure of transmission at the neuromuscular junction (NMJ). Autoantibodies in MG target the acetylcholine receptors (AChRs) as well as non-AChR components like muscle-specific tyrosine kinase (MuSK). Autoantibodies against AChRs are produced by B cells in the germinal centres (GCs), formed in the medulla of MG thymus and circulated to the post-synaptic side of the neuromuscular junction (NMJ) leading to complement-mediated destruction of the post-synaptic folds of NMJ and internalization of AChRs. The incidence and prevalence of MG have increased particularly in elderly, but clinical presentations vary substantially and recognition depends on classic disease phenotype. This chapter focuses on clinical and immunological aspects of MG and its subgroups based on its characterization of the antigenic targets.

Keywords: autoimmune disorders, autoantibodies, myasthenia gravis, acetylcholine receptors, B-cell receptors, cell-based assays, seronegative myasthenia gravis

1. History of myasthenia gravis

Myasthenia gravis (MG) is an autoimmune syndrome caused by the failure of neuromuscular transmission, which results from the binding of autoantibodies to proteins involved in signalling at the neuromuscular junction. Neurobiology of myasthenia gravis states that it is an antibody-mediated autoimmune disorder where antibodies to the acetylcholine receptors (AChR) cause complement-mediated destruction of the post-synaptic folds of the neuromuscular junction (NMJ) and internalisation of AChRs. This results in reduced muscle-nerve synaptic transmission and fatigable muscle weakness, one of the characteristic clinical features, in MG patients. It mainly affects the voluntary muscles including muscles of the neck, eyelids, limb and diaphragm. Antibodies to AChRs and their effects on AChR number and function have been recognized since 45 years. However, their characterization and increasing recognition of antigenic targets added to understand different forms of MG.

Other subgroups of MG includes early-onset MG, late-onset MG, MuSK MG, seronegative MG (SNMG), neonatal MG, depends on the presentation and proteins involved in the disease. Some MG patients do not have detectable antibodies against AChRs and are termed as SNMG. In SNMG, antibodies are directed against the extracellular domain of Musk and inhibit agrin-induced AChR clustering in muscle myotubes [1]. Immunoglobulin G antibodies against Musk have been described in [2] and IgM alters AChR in *in vitro* assays [1].

The incidence and prevalence has increased particularly in older individuals [3, 4]. The yearly incidence has also risen in all studies [5] due to significant increase among older males as well as females [6].

The role of the antibodies that cause myasthenia gravis was clearly established in the 1970s but characterization of antigenic targets evolved till now. Confirmation that antibodies to AChR alone could cause myasthenia gravis, came from immunisation against purified AChRs [7], and the fact that monoclonal antibodies to AChR can produce similar effects in laboratory animals [8]. However they also tested that plasma exchange, removes circulating antibodies, which leads to a substantial but transient improvement in muscle function lasting up to 2 months [9].

2. Diagnostic and clinical classification of MG

Autoantibodies against AChR were present in 85% sera of MG patient [10]. After few years, antibodies against MuSK were reported in 70% of patients with generalized seronegative MG [11]. Approximately 15% of patients with generalized MG do not have AChR antibodies, previously defined as 'seronegative' MG and about 40% of them have antibodies against MuSK; about two-third of the remaining 60% has low-affinity antibodies against AChR undetectable by conventional assays [12, 13]. In MG, 90% of all cases are associated with MuSK and AChR antibodies and are convincingly pathogenic. Besides, some of the antibodies can be associated with special clinical phenotypes. The clinical hallmark of MG is fatigable weakness, involving susceptible muscle groups in the body. It is the most characteristic feature of MG which becomes more evident on exertion and improves with rest. The course of MG is variable. Many patients experience intermittent worsening of symptoms triggered by infections, emotional stress, surgeries or medications, particularly during the first year of the disease.

3. Autoantibodies in MG

Early-onset myasthenia gravis is defined as presenting before age 40 years and is more common in women as per MG Foundation of America. Most are positive for AChR antibodies, and the thymus gland is enlarged. These patients have antibodies to other muscle antigens, but might have other organ-specific autoantibodies [14–16]. Recently, it has been found that, tested serum from EOMG patients, females produced higher amounts of antibodies against clustered AChRs than males. On titration, no significant decrease in level of antibodies was observed. All these observations are summarized in **Table 1** [17].

The targeted antibodies in most MG cases are against the Ach-gated cation channel $\alpha 1$ AChR [18]. Two isoforms of AChR, foetal and adult, differ in the composition of five subunits: the two $\alpha 1$, one δ and one $\beta 1$ subunits, the foetal receptor contains one γ and replaced by one ε subunit in the adult receptor [17]. The main immunogenic region (MIR) is located to the extracellular top of the $\alpha 1$ subunit on the ACh binding site as shown in **Figure 2**. The antibodies against AChRs are mostly complement-fixing IgG1 or IgG3, which recognizes the native conformation easily. The conventional assay to detect AChR antibodies in the sera is radioimmunoprecipitation assay which is based on the mixture of foetal and adult 125I- α –BuTx labelled AChR purified from a human muscle cell line. The sensitivity of the assay is about 80–85% in generalized MG. Alternatively, a non-radioactive cell-based assay (CBA) using cells co-transfected with AChR subunits and rapsyn that clusters AChR at NMJ, detected AChR antibodies in few patients, earlier regarded as 'seronegative' with conventional RIPA [13].

Late-onset myasthenia gravis is defined as its first presentation in people older than 40 years. The thymus gland is not enlarged, but there is an HLA association with B7 and DR2 [17]. Thymoma-associated myasthenia gravis is not age specific, but can be presented at any age and the peak onset is during the 4th– 6th decades. There are no clear HLA associations. The patients usually have antibodies to other muscle antigens such as titin and ryanodine receptor [18].

		Generalised myasthenia gravis(MG) anti-AChR–seropositive (RIA)		
	Ocular MG	**Early-onset (EOMG)**	**Late-onset (LOMG)**	**Thymoma**
Onset-age (years)	4–90	10–45	>45	>10
M:F ratio	3:2	1:3	3:2	1:1
% of all MG	20	20	50	10
HLA/other genes	Not clear	DR3/52a -- B8 PTPN22 TNIP1	DR2/ 51 - B7	Not clear
Autoantibodies	AChR MuSK	AChR	AChR	Musk/AChR/ SN
AChR	+ or –	+++ - +	++	++
MuSK	–	–	–	–
Striated muscle/titin	–	–	++ (70%)	++ (>90%)
Thymic histology	Hyperplasia + or –	Hyperplasia (>80%)	Atrophy	Epithelial neoplasia (+adj. hyperplasia)

Age at onset, gender ratio and other factors in this chart describes clinical basis of Classification 'OF' MG with Clasification 'IN' MG, based on the estimated results on MG serum testing till 2013.

Table 1. Clinical classification of MG.

Ocular myasthenia gravis is restricted to the eye muscles. The titres of antibodies to AChR are lowest in this subgroup, and undetectable in 40–60% of patients. However, electromyography and *in vitro* studies on muscle biopsy samples indicate that the disease is probably present sub-clinically in other muscles [19]. Ocular weakness, presenting as fluctuating ptosis and/or diplopia, is the most common initial presentation of MG, occurring in approximately 85% of patients [20].

MG with thymoma, about 10–15% of patients have thymoma, while 30% of thymomas are associated with MG. Thymoma is equally common in men and women. It can occur at any age, but the peak of onset is around 50 years. Thymoma associated with titin or especially with RyR antibodies may have more severe disease course similar to MuSK-MG, characterized by progressive oropharyngeal weakness. Thymoma is mostly associated with high titer of AChR antibodies. Its symptoms usually persist after thymectomy [21].

3.1. Neonatal MG

Neonatal MG occurs to the babies born to the women having MG regardless of its presentation at the time of pregnancy. It is estimated to be 10% among individuals. It is caused by placental transfer of maternal IgG AChR antibodies. The mothers had very high titres of antibodies specific for the foetal isoform of the AChR, and low concentrations of antibodies directed towards the adult isoform of the AChR (Observations from EOMG patients).

3.2. Anti-Musk MG

Musk is a transmembrane endplate polypeptide involved in a signalling pathway that maintains the normal functional integrity of the NMJ as shown in **Figure 1** [18, 22]. Musk antibodies are mainly IgG4 and are not complement activating, unlike the IgG1 and IgG3 anti-AChR antibodies [26]. Anti-Musk antibodies adversely affect the maintenance of AChR clustering at the muscle endplate, leading to reduced numbers of functional AChRs [20]. Apart from ELISA, a highly sensitive and specific cell-based assay using Musk-transfected HEK cells have been developed and its expression was found very high. Some of the sera of Musk-MG reacted with clustered AChRs as well, showing that low-affinity IgG and IgM antibodies to AChR may be present in a few Musk-MG patients [14]. IgG4 antibodies were previously known in autoimmune disease and thought to occur as a benign phenomenon in conjunction with resolution of allergic reactions. However, they are recognised in other diseases, such as forms of pemphigus [27].

4. Other antibodies

Lrp4 is similarly essential as Musk in the development and function of the adult NMJ, where it performs both anterograde and retrograde signalling roles [24]. These roles highlighted it as a putative antigen of interest, and LRP4 antibodies have been reported in Japanese [28] and European patients. The antibodies were of the complement-activating IgG1 type [28, 29] and impeded agrin-induced clustering of AChRs.

Agrin and collagen Q, antibodies to agrin have been identified in a small number of 'triple negative' MG sera (samples negative for AChR, Musk and LRP4 antibodies) at proportions from 15 to 50%. These antibodies sometimes at low titres were found only with AChR or MuSK antibodies [24]. ColQ tied with MuSK within the synapse, is thought to interact also with Musk. ColQ antibodies were reported in 3–4% of all MG patient sera tested and 1.2–5.5% of the AChR/MuSK/LRP4 negative samples [33].

5. Neuromuscular junction

The NMJ has three basic components, the presynaptic motor nerve terminal, site of acetylcholine synthesis, stored and released. Second is the synaptic space and third is the post-synaptic muscle membrane, which contains the AChRs and the enzyme acetylcholinesterase. Neuromuscular transmission begins with the entry of nerve action potential into the nerve terminal and triggers the release of acetylcholine. Exocytosis of synaptic vesicles containing acetylcholine requires calcium, which enters the depolarised nerve terminal via voltage-gated Ca^{2+} channels. Acetylcholine diffuses across the synaptic cleft and interacts with the AChRs on the post-synaptic side of muscle, leading to depolarisation. The action of acetylcholine

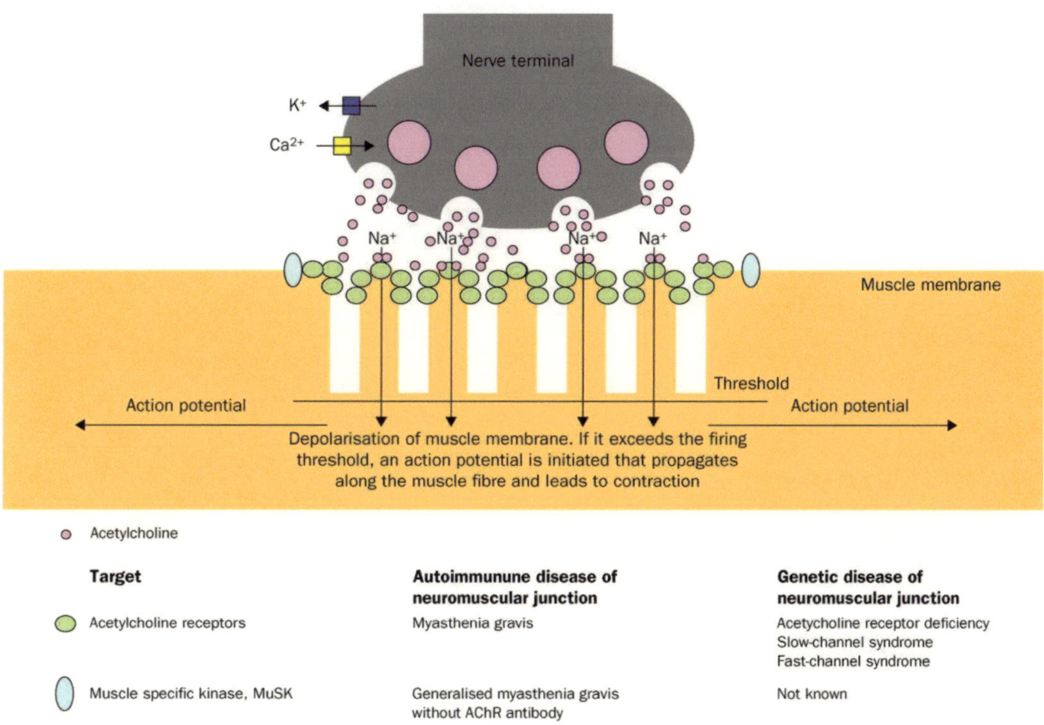

Figure 1. Structure of NMJ, the ion channels involved in neuromuscular transmission and disorders that affect it. The receptor muscle-specific kinase MuSK that now seems to be a major target in AChR seronegative myasthenia gravis is also shown along with other receptors [18].

on the post-synaptic membrane is terminated by acetylcholinesterase. In MG, loss of functional AChRs results in the decrease of threshold required for generation of muscle nerve fibre action potential during repetitive nerve depolarisations, resulting into neuromuscular transmission failure.

6. Structural characterization of AChRs

AChR remains the major antigenic target in MG followed by Musk, LRP4 and agrin. AChR is a pentameric membrane protein consisting of two α, one β, one δ and one ε subunit in the adult muscle, whereas, during development on child birth, the γ subunit takes the place of the ε. These subunits in respective isoforms are organized around a central cation channel. The two binding sites between α and ε or γ and α and δ need to be occupied to be in open state. The main immunogenic region (MIR) is on the extracellular component of each α subunit [13] (**Figure 2**).

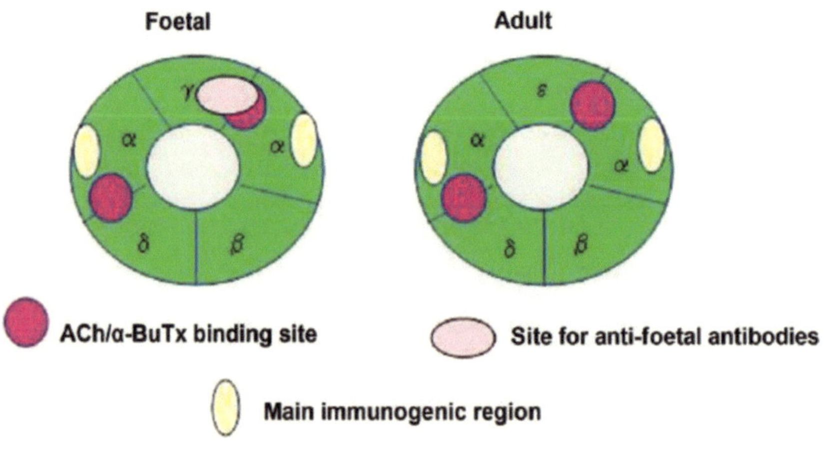

Figure 2. The acetylcholine receptor is a pentameric membrane protein; the membrane consists of five subunits: two α, one β, one δ and either gamma (foetal type) or epsilon (adult type). Acetylcholine and alpha-bungarotoxin bind to sites on the interfaces between the alpha subunit and adjacent subunits. Most of the antibodies in Myasthenia gravis bind to a main immunogenic region on the two α subunits [19].

7. Intra-thymic auto-immune mechanisms in MG

The thymus is an epithelial organ that can be divided into cortex, medulla and cortico-medullary zone. The cortex contains immature lymphocytes alongside epithelial cells and macrophages. The medulla is less cellular containing more mature T lymphocytes, B lymphocytes, epithelial cells, dendritic cells and rare myoid cells. It plays a critical role in self-tolerance with a balance between the generation of T lymphocytes and deletion of auto-reactive T cells, when required [25].

The thymus also has a critical role in AChR Ab+ EOMG patients, having lymphocytic infiltrates in medullary region and germinal centres with distinct areas for B-cell proliferation, differentiation, somatic hypermutation and class switching [25] and thymoma cells do not [23]. Native AChR is also expressed by the myoid cells but are more abundant in hyperplastic thymus [17]. Since a high proportion of patients with MG, demonstrate germinal centre hyperplasia of the thymus or cortical epithelial cell thymoma, the thymus gland was considered a solution to all forms of MG [31]. Whereas, thymectomy is associated with clinical improvement, especially in young patients with thymus hyperplasia and recent disease onset [32].Normally, the thymus functions in early life to prevent autoimmune disorders by its inherent role in clonal deletion by negative selection of auto-reactive T cells and becomes regulatory T cells in early life [33]. Germinal centres normally arise in primary follicles within the secondary lymphoid organs, namely the spleen, lymph nodes and Peyer's patches; these organs provide the necessary microenvironment for the germinal centre response. This justifies the chances for having an autoimmune disorder was not affected by the age of onset of MG. Hence, indicate that acquired and non-genetic factors are involved in the establishment of the immune tolerance breakdown. The clinical impact of exposure to these acquired factors occurs later in life than the clinical impact of thymic involvement [34].

8. Molecular characterization of thymic B cells

Auto-reactive B cells and antibodies can be detected in a variety of neurological diseases. Their causative roles have been established in some disorders and are found to be involved in the pathogenesis of others. During the immune response against an antigen, B cells bearing antigen-specific receptors stimulate to proliferate and differentiate into antibody-secreting plasma cells within the germinal centres. This requires the presence of follicular dendritic cells (FDCs) and activated CD4 T-helper 1(Th-1) cells, CD40/CD40 ligand interaction, and a cocktail of cytokines to create the microenvironment necessary for a germinal centre reaction and a few B cells bearing an appropriate antigen receptors are stimulated to undergo clonal proliferation in the dark zone of the germinal centre and differentiation to centroblasts, centrocytes, memory B cells and plasma cells. Antibody-secreting plasma cells migrate out of the follicle into the surrounding tissue [35].

Several markers on B cells during its proliferation, differentiation and development, characterize them into subsets. CD 20, CD 19, CD 27 and CD 138 which are found on the surface of B cells and plasmablasts, are currently in research to develop B-cell–targeted immunotherapy to treat MG and other related autoimmune neurological disorders.

9. B-cell–directed immunotherapies

Pyridostigmine and corticosteroids plays a central role in the management of MG [36]. Use of azathioprine and other immunosuppressant drugs have been supported to treat MG. Intravenous Immunoglobulin and plasma exchange were also successful treatments for MG.

Rituximab is a chimeric monoclonal antibody directed against the B-cell surface marker CD20. It reduces circulating B-cell counts, and on the basis of its potential for targeting autoreactive B-cell clones, have a therapeutic role in antibody-mediated autoimmune diseases [20]. It has been a useful treatment in IgG4-related diseases which eliminates a population of B or plasma cells responsible for the production of IgG4 antibodies, a targeted B-cell immunotherapy [30].

Ofatumumab is a fully monoclonal anti CD20 antibody which inhibits early B-cell development. Ofatumumab induced enormous depletion of peripheral B lymphocytes in rheumatoid arthritis on the retreatment after rituximab [37]. It has been approved for treating chronic lymphocytic leukaemia. Its effect on development of B cells from MG patients' thymus is currently under study [38–40] . There are several emerging therapies for MG, including tacrolimus, rituximab and antigen-specific apheresis, whereas other treatments await clarification of efficacy and their role in MG. In addition, the complement inhibitory therapy has been shown to be effective in experimental MG [41] and might prove promising in myasthenic crisis and particularly in ocular MG, because of the low expression of complement regulators in extraocular muscle [41].

Recent findings that B cells have critical positive and negative roles in autoimmune disease [42] might lead to particularly effective therapeutic strategies that specifically target anti-AChR antibody-producing memory B cells.

Author details

Kokil Tandon

Address all correspondence to: kokil.tandon@ndcn.ox.ac.uk

Nuffield Department of Clinical Neurosciences, University of Oxford, Oxford, UK; Department of Life Sciences, Brunel University London, Uxbridge, UK

References

[1] Vincent, A., McConville, J., Farrugia, M. E., & Newsom-Davis, J. (2004). Seronegative Myasthenia Gravis. Department of Clinical Neurology, University of Oxford United Kingdom. Seminars in Neurology, 24 (1), 125–133..

[2] Evoli, A., Tonali, A., Padua, L., Monaco, M. L., Scuderi, F., Batocchi, A. P., Marino, M., & Bartoccioni, E. (2003). Clinical correlates with anti-MuSK antibodies in generalized seronegative myasthenia gravis. Brain, 126(Pt 10), 2304–11.

[3] Carr, A. S., Cardwell, C. R., McCarron, P. O., & McConville, J. (2010). A systematic review of population based epidemiological studies in myasthenia gravis. BMC Neurology, 10, 46. doi:101186/1471-2377-10-46

[4] Pakzad, Z., Aziz, T., & Oger, J. (2011). Increasing incidence of myasthenia gravis mong elderly in British Columbia, Canada. Neurology, 76(17), 1526–1528. doi:10.1212/ NL.0b 013e318217e735

[5] Phillips II, L. H., & Torner, J. C. (1996). Epidemiologic evidence for a changing natural history of myasthenia gravis. Neurology, 47(5), 1233–1238.

[6] Poulas, K., Tsibri, E., Kokla, A., Papanastasiou, D., Tsouloufis, T., Marinou, M., et al. (2001). Epidemiology of seropositive myasthenia gravis in Greece. Journal of Neurology, Neurosurgery and Psychiatry, 71(3), 352–356. doi:10.1136/jnnp.71.3.352

[7] Patrick, J., Lindstrom, J. (1973). Autoimmune response to acetylcholine receptor. Science, 180, 871–72.

[8] Lennon, V. A., & Lambert, E. H. (1980). Myasthenia gravis induced by monoclonal antibodies to acetylcholine receptors. Nature, 285(5762), 238–240. doi:10.1038/285238a0

[9] Newsom-Davis, J., Pinching, A. J., Vincent, A., & Wilson, S. G. (1978). Function of circulating antibody to acetylcholine receptor in myasthenia gravis: investigation by plasma exchange. Neurology, 28(3), 266–272.

[10] Lindstrom, J.M., Seybold, M.E., Lennon, V.A., Whittingham, S., Duane, D.D. (1976). Antibody to acetylcholine receptor in myasthenia gravis. Prevalence, clinical correlates, and diagnostic value. Neurology, 26, 1054–1059.

[11] Hoch, W., Mcconville, J., Helms S., Newsom-Davis J., & Vincent, A. M. A (2001). Autoantibodies to the receptor tyrosine kinase MuSK in patients with myasthenia gravis without acetylcholine receptor antibodies. Nature, 7, 1.

[12] Leite, I.M., Jacob, S., Viegas, S., Cossins, J., Clover, L., Morgan, B.P., Beeson, D., Willcox, N., & Vincent, A. (2008). IgG1 antibodies to acetylcholine receptors in "seronegative" myasthenia gravis. Brain, 131, 1940–1952.

[13] Leite, I.M., Waters, P., & Vincent, A. (2010). Diagnostic use of autoantibodies in myasthenia gravis. Autoimmunity, 43, 1–9.

[14] McConville, J., Farrugia, M. E., Beeson, D., Kishore, U., Metcalfe, R., Newsom-Davis, J., et al. (2004). Detection and characterization of MuSK antibodies in seronegative myasthenia gravis. Annals of Neurology, 55(4), 580–584. doi:10.1002/ana.20061

[15] Oosterhuis, H. J. G. H. (1989). The natural course of myasthenia gravis: a long term follow up study. Journal of Neurology, Neurosurgery and Psychiatry, 52(10), 1121–1127.

[16] Kalamida, D., Konstantinos, P., & Auramopoulou, V., et al., (2007). Muscle and neuronal nicotinic acetylcholine receptors: structure, function and pathogenecity. FEBS J, 274, 3799–3845.

[17] Linsdtrom, J., Luo, J., & Kuryatov, A. (2008). Myasthenia gravis and the tops and bottoms of AchRs. Annals of the New York Academy of Sciences, 1132, 29–41.

[18] Vincent, A., Jackie, P, & Jones, D., (2001). Myasthenia gravis. The Lancet, 357(9274), 2122–2128.

[19] Aarli, J. A., Skeie, G. O., Mygland, A., & Guilhus, N. E. Muscle striation antibodies in myasthenia gravis. Diagnostic and functional significance. Annals of Science, 841 (1998), 505–515.

[20] Sommer, N., Melms, A., Weller, M., & Dichens, J. (1993). Ocular myasthenia gravis. A critical review of clinical and pathophysiological aspects. Deaprtment of Neurology, Tübingen University, Germany. Documenta Opthalmologica. Advances in Ophthalmology, 84(4), 309–333.

[21] Matthew, N., Meriggioli, & Sanders, D. B. (2009). Autoimmune myasthenia gravis: emerging clinical and biological heterogeneity. Lancet Neurology, 8(5), 475–490.

[22] Skeie, G. O., & Romi, F. (2008). Paraneoplastic myasthenia gravis: Immunological and clinical aspects. European Journal of Neurology, 15(10), 1029–1033. doi:10.1111/j.1468-1331.2008.02242.

[23] Valenzuela, D. M., Stitt, T. N., DiStefano, P. S., Rojas, E., Mattsson, K., Compton, D. L., et al. (1995). Receptor tyrosine kinase specific for the skeletal muscle lineage: expression in embryonic muscle, at the neuromuscular junction, and after injury. Neuron, 15(3), 573–584. doi:10.1016/0896-6273(95)90146-9

[24] Vincent, A., Newsom-Davis, J., & Batchelor, J. R. (1980). Clinical, pathological, HLA antigen and immunological evidence for disease heterogeneity in myasthenia gravis. Brain, 103, 579–601.

[25] Sims, G. P., Shiono, H., Willcox, N., & Stott, D. I. (2001). Somatic hypermutation and selection of B cells in thymic germinal centers responding to acetylcholine receptor in myasthenia gravis. Journal of Immunology, 167(4), 1935–1944.

[26] Vincent, A. (2008). Autoantibodies in different forms of myasthenia gravis and in the Lambert–Eaton syndrome. Handbook of Clinical Neurology,91, 213–227.

[27] Binks S, Vincent A, Palace J. Myasthenia gravis: a clinical-immunological update. Review. J Neurol. 2016 Apr;263(4):826–34

[28] Pal, J., Rozsa, C., Komoly, S., & Illes, Z. (2011). Clinical and biological heterogeneity of autoimmune myasthenia gravis. Journal of Neuroimmunology, 231(1–2), 43–54.

[29] Parr, J. R., Andrew, M. J., Finnis, M., Beeson, D., Vincent, A., & Jayawant, S. (2014). How common is childhood myasthenia? The UK incidence and prevalence of autoimmune and congenital myasthenia. Archives of Disease in Childhood, 99(6), 539–542. doi:10.1136/archdischild-2013-304788

[30] Huijbers, M. G., Querol, L. A., Niks, E. H., Plomp, J. J., van der Maarel, S. M., Graus, F., et al. (2015). The expanding field of IgG4-mediated neurological autoimmune disorders. European Journal of Neurology, 22(8), 1151–1161. doi:10.1111/ene.12758.

[31] Higuchi, O., Hamuro, J., Motomura, M., et al. (2011). Autoantibodies to low-density lipoprotein receptor–related protein 4 in Myasthenia Gravis. Annals of Neurology, 69(2), 418–422. doi: 10.1002/ana.22312.

[32] Pevzner, A., Schoser, B., Peters, K., et al. (2012). Anti-LRP4 autoantibodies in AChR- and MuSK-antibody negative myasthenia gravis. Journal of Neurology, 259(3), 427–435. doi: 10.1007/s00415-011-6194-7.

[33] Katarzyna, M., Belaya, K., Leite, M., et al. (2015). Collagen Q—a potential target for autoantibodies in myasthenia gravis. Journal of Neurology Science, 348(1–2), 241–244. doi: 10.1016/j.jns.2014.12.015.

[34] Levinson, A. I., & Wheatley, L. M. (1996). The thymus and the pathogenesis of myasthenia gravis. Clinical Immunology and Immunopathology, 78(1), 1–5. doi:10.1006/clin.1996.0001.

[35] Olanow, C. W., Wechsler, S., Sirotkin-Roses, M., Stajich, J., & Roses, A. D. (1987). Thymectomy as primary therapy in myasthenia gravis. Annals of the New York Academy of Sciences, 505, 595–606.

[36] Shevach, E. M. (2000). Regulatory T cells in autoimmmunity. Annual Review of Immunology, 18, 423–449. doi:10.1146/annurev.immunol.18.1.423.

[37] Karni, A., Asmail, A., Drory, V.E., Kolb, H., & Kesler, A. (2016). Thymus involvement in myasthenia gravis: epidemiological and clinical impacts of different self-tolerance breakdown mechanisms. 298:58—62.

[38] Stott, D.I., Hiepe, F., Hummel, M., Steinhauser, G., & Berek, C. (1998). Antigen-driven clonal proliferation of B cells within the target tissue of an autoimmune disease: the salivary glands of patients with Sjögren's syndrome. Journal of Clinical Investigation, 102(5), 938946.

[39] Kawaguchi, N. (2011). Immunosuppressive/immunomodulating therapies in myasthenia gravis-at present and in the near future. Brain and Nerve, 63(7), 737–743.

[40] Quattrocchi, E., Østergaard, M., Taylor, P. C., Van Vollenhoven, R. F., Chu, M., Mallett, S., et al. (2016). Safety of repeated open-label treatment courses of intravenous ofatumumab, a human anti-CD20 monoclonal antibody, in rheumatoid arthritis: results from three clinical trials. PLoS One, 11(6) doi:10.1371/journal.pone.0157961.

[41] Kaminski, H. J., Li, Z., Richmonds, C., Lin, F., & Medof, M. E. (2004). Complement regulators in extraocular muscle and experimental autoimmune myasthenia gravis. Experimental Neurology, 189(2), 333–342. doi:10.1016/j.expneurol.2004.06.005.

[42] Matsushita, T., Yanaba, K., Bouaziz, J. Fujimoto, M., & Tedder, T. F. (2008). Regulatory B cells inhibit EAE initiation in mice while other B cells promote disease progression. Journal of Clinical Investigation, 118(10), 3420–3430. doi:10.1172/JCI36030.

Chapter 8

The Roles of the TNF-Family Member B-Cell Activation Factor Belonging to the TNF-Family (BAFF) in Autoimmunity

Kouichi Hirayama and Miho Nagai

Additional information is available at the end of the chapter

http://dx.doi.org/10.5772/66767

Abstract

The tumor necrosis factor superfamily (TNFSF) member and cytokine known as B-cell activation factor belonging to the TNF-family (BAFF) has been identified as one of the key factors in the selection and survival of B cells. Overexpression of BAFF in mice leads to autoimmunity, whereas BAFF-deficient mice lack mature B cells. Although under normal concentrations of BAFF, non–self-reactive B cells survived and autoreactive B cells were deleted, a higher concentration of BAFF contributed to the survival of autoreactive B cells and elevated autoantibody production. Lupus-prone mice have increased serum levels of BAFF during the onset and progression of disease. The serum BAFF levels are elevated in patients with autoimmune diseases, such as systemic lupus erythematosus, rheumatoid arthritis, Sjögren's syndrome and ANCA-associated vasculitis, and showed positive correlations with autoantibodies. Based on the development of autoimmune disorders in animal models of BAFF overexpression and the elevated levels of serum BAFF in patients with autoimmune diseases, it appears that BAFF may be associated with autoimmune processes and that BAFF may be a potential biomarker for disease activity in autoimmune diseases. BAFF may also be important as a therapeutic target in those diseases and several BAFF-neutralizing agents are currently undergoing clinical trials.

Keywords: B-cell activation factor belonging to the TNF-family, systemic lupus erythematosus, rheumatoid arthritis, Sjögren's syndrome, systemic vasculitis, belimumab, atacicept

1. Introduction

B cells are associated with autoimmune diseases (in functions such as the production of pathogenic autoantibodies) and with multiple pathogenic functions such as autoantigen uptake and transport, autoantigen presentation to T cells, the production of humoral factors and migration to sites of inflammation. As one of the key factors in the selection and survival of B cells, a closely related cytokine of the tumor necrosis factor (TNF) superfamily (TNFSF) was identified, i.e., the B-cell activation factor belonging to the TNF-family (BAFF). Here we review the physiology of BAFF and its receptors, the roles of BAFF and the effects of BAFF blockade in autoimmune diseases.

2. The basic characteristics of BAFF

2.1. BAFF and its receptors

BAFF (also known as B-lymphocyte stimulator) is a member of the TNF superfamily 13B (TNFSF13B) of proteins that regulate immune responses [1, 2]. The gene for BAFF is located on human chromosome 13q34 and on mouse chromosome 8 [3]. BAFF exists in two forms, a membrane-bound form and a soluble form. Membrane-bound BAFF can be released from cells via proteolytic cleavage from a furin protease site by metalloproteases and released in a soluble form [4].

Soluble BAFF mainly exists in the form of homotrimers. An *in vitro* study showed that 20 BAFF trimers may associate to form a multimeric BAFF 60-mer (which exhibits a virus-like structure) at a neutral or alkaline pH; at an acidic pH, the BAFF 60-mer dissociates into BAFF trimers [5]. However, whether soluble BAFF does or does not form BAFF 60-mer *in vivo* is a controversial question [6]. BAFF is expressed on the surface of many cell types, including antigen-presenting cells (B cells, monocytes, macrophages, dendritic cells) [7, 8], neutrophils [9] and activated T cells [10]. BAFF mRNA has also been detected in bone marrow-derived stromal cells, astrocytes and fibroblast-like synoviocytes in response to proinflammatory cytokines [11].

Soluble BAFF binds to three receptors that are present on several immune cell types—i.e., BAFF-receptor (BAFF-R; also known as BR3 and TNF-receptor superfamily 13C), transmembrane activator and calcium modulator and cyclophilin-ligand interactor (TACI; also known as TNF-receptor superfamily 13B) and B-cell maturation antigen (BCMA; also known as TNF-receptor superfamily 17)—at various times during their differentiation [1]. BCMA is expressed on transitional type 1 (T1) cells [12] and on plasma cells [13, 14], whereas TACI and BAFF-R are expressed on innate immune B cells (marginal zone B cells and transitional type 2 [T2] B cells) and mature B cells [12].

A proliferation-inducing ligand (APRIL), which is a member of the TNFSF (TNFSF13A), was identified as the homologous molecule of BAFF [15]. The gene for APRIL is located on human chromosome 17p13.1 and on mouse chromosome 11 [16]. Similar to soluble BAFF, soluble APRIL exists mainly in the form of homotrimers. APRIL differs from BAFF in that APRIL is not present on the cell surface. APRIL is processed by the Golgi apparatus, which involves cleavage at the furin protease site and the resulting soluble APRIL is released from the cell [17]. Although APRIL trimers are unable to form a multimeric 60-mer, APRIL trimers bind to heparan sulfate proteoglycans (HSPGs) and the binding of multiple APRIL to HSPGs enhances local APRIL signaling [18]. Moreover, HSPGs provide a platform for APRIL multimerization, which promotes the occurrence of APRIL multimerization [19].

Thus, the BAFF system involves two ligands (BAFF and APRIL) and three receptors (BAFF-R, TACI and BCMA) and the ligands take three forms (membrane-bound, soluble homotrimers and the multimeric form) (**Figure 1**) [1]. However, APRIL binds to TACI and BCMA but not to BAFF-R [20]. Membrane-bound BAFF and the multimeric BAFF 60-mer binds to BAFF-R, TACI and BCMA, whereas the soluble homotrimers BAFF binds to only BAFF-R [20, 21]. BAFF-R is expressed on resting, marginal zone and germinal center B cells and TACI is expressed on mature B cells and plasma cells [20, 21]. BCMA was identified prior to BAFF-R as a receptor for BAFF [22, 23], but its expression is restricted to germinal center B cells, memory B cells and plasma cells [24–26]. BCMA is a high-affinity receptor for APRIL, whereas in humans BCMA binds BAFF with low affinity.

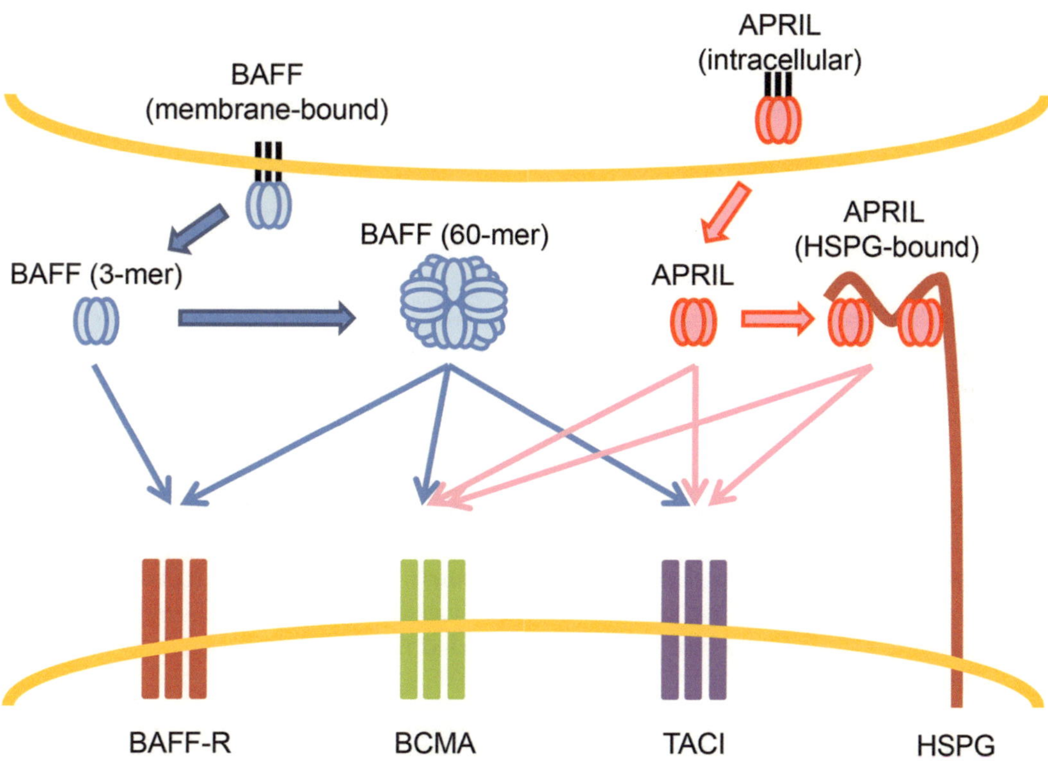

Figure 1. The BAFF system involves two ligands (BAFF and APRIL) and three receptors (BAFF-R, TACI and BCMA) and the ligands take three forms (membrane-bound, soluble homotrimers and the multimeric form).

2.2. Functions of BAFF

The B cells differentiate from hematopoietic stem cells to pro-B cells, pre-B cells, immature B cells, T1 B cells, T2 B cells, mature B cells, activated B cells, memory B cells and plasma cells sequentially and the interaction of BAFF with BAFF-R is essential for the survival of T2 B cell [1, 22, 27]. Increased competition for BAFF results in a deletion of autoreactive B cells, whereas decreased competition for BAFF in the context of B-cell lymphopenia or increased levels of circulating BAFF results in a relaxation of the B-cell selection and a release of more autoreactive naïve B cells. BAFF-R is upregulated by B-cell receptor (BCR) ligation on mature B cells [28] and is expressed on resting memory B cells [14].

However, it is clear that the survival and reactivation of B-cell memory is BAFF-independent. BAFF-R mediates most BAFF-dependent functions in the naïve B-cell population [29], whereas BCMA is needed for the optimal generation of long-lived plasma cells [30]. Survival of plasma cells expressing TACI and/or BCMA depends on either BAFF or APRIL secreted by dendritic cells and monocyte/macrophages in the lymph node or bone marrow [31]. In contrast, peritoneal B1 cells do not require BAFF or APRIL for their survival [1].

BAFF also plays an important role in immunoglobulin production and class switching. T cell-independent type II responses require the interaction of multimeric BAFF 60-mer or membrane-bound BAFF with TACI [32–34]. TACI-deficient mice have decreased serum IgM and decreased IgM responses to T-independent antigens, but they have increased B-cell numbers and develop an autoimmune phenotype [35]. BAFF induces the CD40-independent immunoglobulin-class switching through the interaction of B cells and the dendritic cells; human dendritic cells upregulate BAFF and APRIL induced immunoglobulin-class switch from $C\mu$ to $C\gamma$ and/or $C\alpha$ genes in B cells in the presence of IL-10 and TGF-β and in the presence of IL-4, BAFF and APRIL-induced immunoglobulin-class switch from $C\mu$ to $C\varepsilon$ [35]. IgG responses are much less BAFF-dependent and class-switching to IgA appears to be dependent upon the interaction of APRIL, multimerized by proteoglycans, with TACI [36, 37].

BAFF is an essential component of the innate-immune response and is induced in myeloid dendritic cells by type I interferons (IFNs) [38]. BAFF upregulates toll-like receptor (TLR) expression, promotes B-cell survival and promotes immunoglobulin class-switching and plasma cell differentiation together with interleukin (IL-6) [39, 40]. The activation of TLR-9 in B cells by oligodeoxynucleotides containing CpG motifs upregulates the expression of TACI and increases BCR-mediated signaling [39, 41]. In contrast, the activation of TLR-4 in B cells by lipopolysaccharides upregulates BAFF-R and induces the activated B cells to become susceptible to Fas/CD95-mediated apoptosis [42].

2.3. BAFF-R signaling

Membrane proximal signaling by BAFF-R has been attributed to the TNFR-associated factor (TRAF) molecules, which bind directly or via adapter molecules to intracellular domains of TNFRSF members [43, 44]. Although only TRAF3 binds BAFF-R directly [45, 46], signaling occurs via the concerted actions of TRAF2 and TRAF3, which negatively regulate the receptor [43]. Thus, mice lacking TRAF2 or TRAF3 exhibit a phenotype consistent with BAFF transgenic mice and can persist *in vitro* in the absence of survival factors as well as *in vivo* in the absence of BAFF [47–50]. On the other hand, the inactivation of TRAF3 also allowed for the formation and maintenance of the marginal zone B-cell compartment [49, 50], indicating that both BAFF-dependent survival and differentiation signals are dependent upon TRAF2/TRAF3. TRAF2 and TRAF3 are recruited, leading to the release of NF-κB-inducing kinase (NIK), which phosphorylates IKK1, leading to p100 processing to p52 and the activation of NF-κB (**Figure 2**).

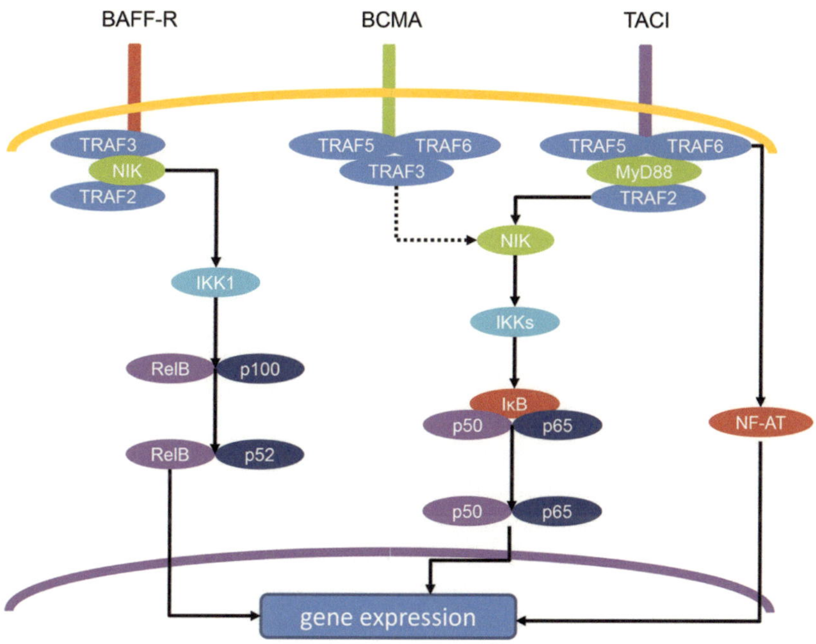

Figure 2. Signaling of three BAFF receptors (BAFF-R, TACI and BCMA).

TACI intracellular domain interacted with TRAF2, TRAF5 and TRAF6 and these interactions induce NF-κB and JNK activations [51, 52]. On the other hand, in immunoglobulin class-switch signaling, TACI can activate NF-κB in the myeloid differentiation primary response protein 88 (MyD88)/the interleukin-1 receptor-associated kinase 4 (IRAK4)-dependent manner similar to TLR signaling [53]. MyD88 and TRAF2 bind to the same region of TACI and acts cooperatively to activate NF-κB [53]. BCMA, BAFF-R and CD40 do not share the ability to bind MyD88.

BCMA-deficient mice have normal B-cell development and the life span of mutant B lymphocytes is comparable to that of wild-type B cells [54]. Moreover, the humoral immune responses of BCMA-deficient mice to T-cell-independent and -dependent antigens were also intact [54]. However, in BCMA-deficient mice, the reduced number of long-lived IgG-producing bone marrow plasma cells was demonstrated compared with wild-type mice [13] and BCMA may be the receptor on plasma cells critical for plasma cell survival. An overexpression of BCMA in human embryonic kidney 293 cells activated canonical NF-κB signaling and coimmunoprecipitation studies indicated that BCMA could interact with NIK and the

IKK complex [55, 56]. Consistently, the survival of long-lived plasma cells does not require BAFF but is dependent upon APRIL [18, 57]. Thus, much remains to be known regarding BCMA signaling by APRIL/BAFF in terminally differentiated plasma cells.

3. BAFF in autoimmune diseases

3.1. Animal models

3.1.1. BAFF-deficient or transgenic models

Mice deficient in BAFF lack T2 B cells, mature marginal zone and follicular B cells and have significantly reduced spleen weights, whereas B-cell differentiation and/or proliferation in bone marrow, T1 B cells and other hematopoietic cell lineages appear normal [22, 58]. BAFF-deficient mice have a reduction in the total serum immunoglobulin level and show diminished T cell-independent and T cell-dependent antibody responses [22, 58]. On the other hand, the phenotypes of BAFF-, BCMA-, TACI- and BAFF-R-deficient mice clearly indicate that the BAFF survival signal in transitional and mature B cells is mediated by BAFF-R in mice and not through BCMA and TACI [22, 34, 54, 58, 59].

Mice transgenic (Tg) for BAFF have vastly increased numbers of mature B and effector T cells and they develop autoimmune-like manifestations such as the presence of high levels of rheumatoid factors (RFs), circulating immune complexes, anti-DNA autoantibodies and immunoglobulin deposition in the kidneys, closely mimicking human systemic lupus erythematosus (SLE) and Sjögren's syndrome (SjS) [47, 60, 61]. These Tg mice showed also severe enlargement of the spleen, lymph nodes and Peyer's patches because of an increased number of B220 cells and hypergammaglobulinemia contributed by elevations of serum IgM, IgG, IgA and IgE was observed [61].

Older BAFF-Tg mice demonstrate characteristics of SjS, such as enlarged salivary glands due to inflammation and leukocytic infiltrates and reduced saliva production as a consequence of acinar cell destruction [62]. BAFF induced the survival of a subset of splenic immature B cells, referred to as T2 B cells [63]. BAFF treatment allowed T2 B cells to survive and differentiate into mature B cells in response to signals through the B-cell receptor (BCR) [63]. The T2 and the marginal zone B-cell compartments were particularly enlarged in BAFF Tg mice [63].

Immature transitional B cells are targets for negative selection, a feature thought to promote self-tolerance [63]. Although BAFF overexpression did not affect the development of self-reactive B cells normally deleted in the bone marrow or during the early stages of peripheral development, BAFF overexpression rescued from deletion of selfreactive B cells, which normally deleted around the late T2 stage of peripheral development [64]. Moreover, self-reactive B cells normally selectively deleted from the marginal zone repopulated this compartment by BAFF overexpression [64]. This partial subversion of B-cell self-tolerance is likely to underlie the autoimmunity associated with BAFF overexpression (**Figure 3**).

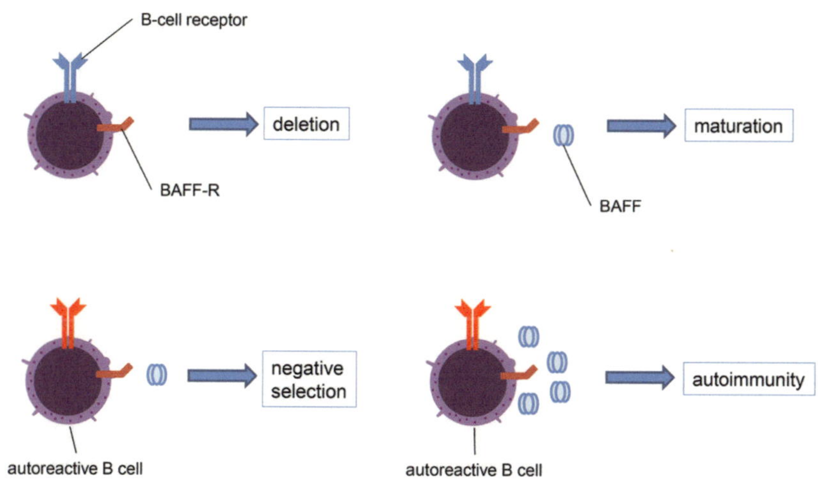

Figure 3. The associations B-cell maturation or B-cell self-tolerance and BAFF expressions.

3.1.2. Animal models of autoimmune diseases

In two murine models of human SLE, MRL/Mp-lpr/lpr and NZB/W F1 mice, there are increased serum levels of BAFF that seem to correlate with autoimmune kidney damage [60]. In NZB/W F1 mice, treatment with soluble TACI-Ig fusion protein inhibits the development of proteinuria and prolongs survival of these mice [60]. In BXSB murine lupus model, treatment with soluble fusion protein consisting of human BAFF-R and human mutant IgG4 Fc resulted in significant reduction in peripheral and splenic B-cells and in proteinuria [65]. In SLE-prone NZM 2328 mice deficient in BAFF, serum autoantibody levels and glomerular IgG and C3 depositions were significantly reduced compared with wild-type NZM 2328 mice [66] and those clinical and pathological responses were more resistant to disease-promoting properties of IFN-α [67].

3.2. Human autoimmune diseases

Similar to BAFF-R-deficient mice, humans with the BAFF-R gene deletion have severe B-cell lymphopenia. B cells are arrested at the transitional B-cell stage and this condition presents with adult-onset antibody-deficiency syndrome [68]. Humans with this condition have diminished numbers of mature B cells, e.g., follicular, marginal zone and memory B cells and their T-independent immune responses are severely impaired.

In relation to the possible role of BAFF in autoimmunity, patients with autoimmune diseases such as SLE, RA, SjS and antineutrophil cytoplasmic antibody (ANCA)-associated vasculitis (AAV) have all been shown to have elevated levels of BAFF.

3.2.1. Systemic lupus erythematosus

The BAFF levels of 110 plasma samples and 40 serum samples from 150 SLE patients were found to be elevated compared to the samples from 40 normal controls [69]. In that study, the

SLE patients with high levels of BAFF exhibited significantly higher levels of antidouble-strand-DNA antibody in each of the IgG, IgM and IgA classes compared to the SLE patients with low levels of BAFF and the normal controls [69]. In a study of serum BAFF levels in 185 patients with various systemic immune-based rheumatic diseases (including 95 with SLE, 67 with RA, 23 with other diseases), serum BAFF levels were elevated in 21% of the 185 patients and those levels in the SLE patients correlated with the antidouble-strand-DNA antibody titers [70].

In a longitudinal study of serum BAFF levels in 68 SLE patients, the serum BAFF levels were persistently or intermittently elevated in 50% of the patients and the blood BAFF mRNA levels were also elevated in 61% of the patients [71]. In SLE patients with elevated serum BAFF levels, treatments with high-dose corticosteroids led to a marked reduction of the serum BAFF levels [71]. Regarding the association of serum BAFF levels with disease activity, those levels were correlated with not only antidouble-strand-DNA antibody titers but also the safety of estrogens in lupus erythematosus: National Assessment (SELENA) version of the systemic lupus erythematosus disease activity index (SLEDAI) score in 245 patients with SLE [72].

Of the peripheral blood mononuclear cells (PBMCs) from normal controls, only CD14+ cells (monocytes) expressed surface BAFF and this expression tended to be very modest, whereas the level of BAFF expression was frequently increased in PBMCs from SLE patients and some CD14− cells as well as CD14+ cells were present [71]. In another SLE cohort of 60 patients, the peripheral blood leukocyte levels of BAFF mRNA were correlated with the serum BAFF protein levels and the BAFF mRNA levels were more closely associated with serum immunoglobulin levels and SLEDAI scores than were the serum BAFF protein levels [73]. In 75 SLE patients, elevated serum BAFF and elevated PBMC BAFF mRNA levels in active SLE patients were observed compared with those in stable SLE patients and controls and those levels in active SLE patients with proteinuria were higher than those in active SLE patients without proteinuria [74].

BAFF-R expressions on CD27−CD38low (resting naïve) and CD27+CD38low (resting memory) B cells were equivalent between SLE patients and controls, but those expressions on CD38+ (germinal center) B cells and CD27+CD38++ (plasmablast) cells were reduced compared to controls [75]. The occupancy of BAFF-R on B cells from SLE patients would render them less responsive to exogenous BAFF [75]. BAFF-R expressions on CD19+IgD+CD27−, CD19+IgD+CD27+ and CD19+IgD−CD27+ B cells in SLE patients were reduced compared to controls [76]. Decreased BAFF-R expressions on CD19+ B cells were more obvious in SLE patients with nephritis, whereas the expression of TACI on CD19+ B cells in lupus nephritis was upregulated [76].

BAFF-R expressions on CD19+ B cells were correlated with negative SLEDAI scores [76], but TACI expression in CD19+ B cells was positively correlated positively with the SLEDAI score [77]. The expression of BAFF-R on CD19+ cells (B cells) in active SLE patients was downregulated compared to those in stable SLE patients and controls and the expression of BAFF-R on CD19+ cells was negatively correlated with serum BAFF levels and BAFF mRNA levels in PBMCs [74]. Thus, elevated BAFF in serum and PBMCs and a reduced expression of BAFF-R and overexpression of TACI on B cells were demonstrated in SLE.

http://dx.doi.org/10.5772/66767

3.2.2. Rheumatoid arthritis

It was demonstrated that serum BAFF levels in 67 rheumatoid arthritis (RA) patients were higher than those in 48 normal controls and elevated serum BAFF levels were correlated with serum IgG levels and RF titers in 42 RA patients [70]. The serum BAFF levels in 53 patients with RA were higher than those in 39 healthy controls, but lower than those in 41 patients with Sjögren's syndrome [62]. In 129 patients with autoimmune diseases including 28 RA patients, elevated serum levels of BAFF correlated with RF titers [78]. Elevated serum BAFF levels were observed in an early RA stage: serum BAFF levels were higher in 48 early RA patients (disease duration <1 year) compared to 48 patients with rheumatic disease other than RA or 50 healthy controls, but not 49 patients with longstanding RA (disease duration >1 year) [79]. In 48 early-RA patients, the serum BAFF levels correlated with IgG-, IgA- and IgM-RF titers and anti-CCP antibody levels [79]. Thus, serum BAFF levels were elevated in RA patients and those levels were associated with autoantibodies, including RF titers.

Synovial fluid levels of BAFF in RA patients were more elevated than the serum BAFF levels in the same patients and the synovial fluid and serum BAFF levels were correlated with each other [80]. The synovial fluid levels of BAFF in RA patients were also correlated with monocyte, lymphocyte, neutrophil and total nucleated cell counts [80]. In mononuclear cells extracted from the synovium of RA patients, BAFF and BAFF mRNA were expressed on B cells, T cells and monocytes [81]. In that study, BAFF was not expressed on the surface of fibroblast-like synoviocytes (FLSs) extracted from the synovium of RA patients, but BAFF mRNA was detected in FLSs [81]. There was no difference in BAFF mRNA of FLSs from the synovial tissue of RA patients compared with those from patients with osteoarthritis and the normal controls, but the BAFF mRNA of those cells was enhanced by IFN-γ or TNF-α [82]. In cocultures of peripheral B cells with FLSs from synovial tissue of RA patients, the expression of RAG genes—which could induce a revision of the B-cell receptor genes, resulting in autoreactivity—was induced in peripheral B cells by BAFF and IL-6 [83]. Moreover, a BAFF-dependent class switch recombination was demonstrated in the coculture of peripheral B cells with FLSs from synovial tissue of RA patients [84]. These findings suggested that the overexpression of BAFF may be associated with autoimmunity at sites of inflammation in RA.

There was no difference in the BAFF-R expression on peripheral naïve B (CD19+CD27−) and memory B (CD19+CD27+) cells among RA patients before treatment, RA patients during remission and normal controls, but the BAFF-R expression on both types of B cells in RA patients at relapse was significantly lower than that in the RA patients before treatment and the normal controls [85]. Although the BAFF-R expressions on PBMCs and B cells were reduced, BAFF-R in synovial tissues from RA patients was highly expressed [86].

However, in another study, the BAFF-R expression on peripheral B cells increased with disease progression (very early, early and established RA) and the TACI expression on peripheral B cells increased in all stages of RA patients [87]. Thus, elevated BAFF in serum and synovial tissue of RA was demonstrated, but the BAFF-R expression varied.

3.2.3. *Sjögren's syndrome*

It was demonstrated that serum BAFF levels in 41 patients with SjS were higher than those in 53 SLE patients, 53 RA patients and 39 healthy controls [62]. In the investigation of both serum BAFF and APRIL, in a comparison with six healthy donors the serum levels of both BAFF and APRIL in 29 SjS patients were elevated, but compared with SjS patients without anti-SSA antibody, only the serum APRIL levels in the SjS patients with anti-SSA antibody were elevated [88].

Although the serum BAFF levels failed to correlate with anti-SSA antibody, anti- SSB antibody or RF in those studies, several other studies demonstrated that the serum BAFF levels correlated with autoantibodies [78, 89, 90]. In 49 patients with SjS, elevated serum levels of BAFF were demonstrated compared to those in 47 healthy controls and there was a strong correlation between the serum BAFF levels and anti-SSA antibodies and RF levels [89]. In 129 patients with autoimmune diseases including 58 SjS patients, elevated serum levels of BAFF in the SjS group were correlated with anti-SSA antibody [78]. In an investigation of 127 SjS patients, elevated serum levels of BAFF in SjS correlated with anti-SSA and anti-SSB antibodies [90]. Serum BAFF levels in SjS patients with hypergammaglobulinemia were also elevated compared to those of patients with normal IgG levels [91].

The serum BAFF levels in SjS patients with the formation of ectopic germinal centers were elevated compared to those of patients without ectopic germinal centers [92]. BAFF mRNA expression and production in circulating monocytes and T cells from SjS patients by IFN-α stimulation were higher than those from normal controls [93]. The expression of BAFF and its mRNA were also demonstrated in T cells infiltrating labial salivary glands of biopsy specimens from SjS patients [94]. In salivary glands, BAFF expressions were also observed in IFN-stimulated salivary gland epithelial cells [95] and infiltrating B cells [96]. These findings suggested that BAFF may be associated with the immunopathogenesis of SjS.

Unstimulated peripheral monocytes from 13 SjS patients produced higher amounts of BAFF and IL-6 compared to those of 12 healthy donors [97]. In that study, the expressions of BAFF-R and transcription factors regulating IL-6 in monocytes from SjS patients were also elevated. Thus, BAFF may also be associated with monocyte activation.

Although elevated BAFF in serum and salivary glands of SjS patients were demonstrated, the BAFF-R expression varied. The expression of BAFF-R on peripheral B cells in 20 SjS patients was decreased compared to that in 15 controls and there was no difference in BAFF-R mRNA levels of B cells between SjS patients and controls [98]. On the other hand, in a study of BAFF-R expression in the salivary glands, the expression of BAFF-R on B cells was observed, but the expressions of TACI and BCMA were not [96].

Serum BAFF levels differed among SjS patients with and without lymphoproliferative disorders (lymphoma or prelymphomatous manifestations): higher levels of serum BAFF in 42 SjS patients with lymphoproliferative disorders were demonstrated compared to those in 34 SjS patients without these disorders [99]. A higher frequency of the minor T allele of the rs9514828 BAFF polymorphism in the high-risk SjS group for lymphoma was demonstrated [100]. Moreover, in SjS patients with younger-age onset (at <40 years old), the generalized odds ratio for the development of mucosa-associated tissue lymphoma was 6.1 in the presence of the BAFF-R His159Tyr mutation [101]. These findings suggested that BAFF may also associated with an increased risk of progression to lymphoma.

3.2.4. *ANCA-associated vasculitis*

Several studies of serum BAFF levels in AAV patients have been reported. It was demonstrated that the serum BAFF levels in 46 granulomatosis with polyangiitis (GPA) patients were significantly elevated compared to those of 62 healthy controls [102]. Elevated serum BAFF levels were observed in untreated GPA patients, but that level in corticosteroid-treated GPA patients was approximately the same as in the healthy controls. Similarly, elevated serum BAFF levels were observed in 87 patients with proteinase-3 (PR3)-AAV compared to the levels of 31 healthy controls, but the BAFF levels in relapsed patients did not differ from those in patients without relapse [103]. In a study of 22 GPA patients, serum BAFF levels were correlated independently and inversely with PR3-ANCA levels, but did not correlate with clinical parameters, i.e., the Birmingham vasculitis activity score (BVAS), the vasculitis damage index (VDI) and the disease extent index (DEI) and with the serum C-reactive protein (CRP) level [104]. Thus, serum BAFF levels in GPA were elevated, but the association between the BAFF level and the PR3-ANCA titer was not established.

Among three types of AAV (41 patients with GPA, 16 patients with microscopic polyangiitis [MPA] and four patients with eosinophilic GPA), elevated serum levels of BAFF were observed only in GPA patients [105]. However, several studies demonstrated that serum BAFF levels were elevated in MPA patients [106, 107]. In myeloperoxidase (MPO)-AAV, the serum BAFF levels in 23 active vasculitis patients were higher than those in 24 inactive vasculitis patients, 13 inactive vasculitis patients with infectious complication and 20 controls [106]. Moreover, there were significant positive correlations between the serum levels of BAFF and the BVAS results, the serum CRP levels and the MPO-ANCA titers.

Similar to those findings, in a study of 121 patients with MPO-AAV (100 of whom had MPA, 18 had GPA and three had renal-limited vasculitis), the serum BAFF levels were significantly elevated in both the patients with active disease and those in remission compared to healthy controls, although the patients with active disease still had significantly higher levels than those in remission. In that study, the serum BAFF levels correlated well with the BVAS results and the erythrocyte sedimentation rate (ESR), but they did not correlate with the MPO-ANCA titer [107]. Thus, serum BAFF levels in MPA were elevated, but the association between the BAFF level and the MPO-ANCA titer was not clear.

In an *in vitro* study of BAFF expression and release in stimulated neutrophils, treatment with PR3-ANCA-IgG significantly increased BAFF expression in neutrophils compared to the expression in untreated and normal IgG-treated cells [108]. Supernatants from PR3-ANCA-IgG-stimulated neutrophils were shown to contain increased levels of BAFF compared to those from untreated and normal IgG-treated neutrophils [108]. Supernatants from neutrophils treated with PR3-ANCA but not normal IgG induced an increase in the cell viability of a B-cell line [108]. In a study of the *in vitro* IgG production in stimulated PBMCs from GPA patients, IL-21 enhanced the production of IgG, whereas stimulation with BAFF alone did not result in increased IgG production [109]. However, the combination of BAFF and IL-21 increased the IgG production more than IL-21 alone [109].

The combination of BAFF and IL-21 induced a significant enhancement in PR3-ANCA production in PBMCs isolated from ANCA-positive patients in comparison with ANCA-negative patients [109]. The stimulatory effect on IgG and PR3-ANCA production by BAFF and IL-21 was further enhanced by the addition of exogenous factors (oligodeoxynucleotides containing CpG motifs) [110]. These findings suggested that elevated BAFF may be associated with ANCA production by autoreactive B-cell survival.

Decreased expression of BAFF-R on circulating B cells and decreased expression of TACI on circulating memory B cells were demonstrated [110]. In another study, there was no difference in soluble TACI levels among active MPO-AAV patients, inactive MPO-AAV patients and controls [111]. On the other hand, in a histological study of biopsy samples from eight patients with GPA, activated B cells in nasal mucosa were located alongside PR3-expressing cells and BAFF-producing cells and BAFF-R-expressing B cells were also identified in the nasal mucosa [112]. The expression of BCMA on plasma cells, lymphocytic and fibroblast-like cells in sinonasal biopsy specimens from GPA patients were elevated, compared to those from nonautoimmune inflammatory rhinosinusitis [113]. In this study, TACI-expressed cells displaying plasma-cell-like morphology were present in sinonasal biopsy specimens from only GPA patients [112]. Although elevated serum BAFF in AAV was demonstrated by several investigations, further studies of BAFF-R in AAV were needed.

3.2.5. Other autoimmune diseases

In addition to systemic autoimmune diseases, the serum BAFF level is also elevated in organ-specific autoimmune diseases. Antiglomerular basement membrane (GBM) disease is an autoimmune disease characterized by the presence of anti-GBM autoantibodies. The most common clinical features include rapidly progressive glomerulonephritis and/or alveolar hemorrhage (goodpasture disease). The serum levels of BAFF in patients with anti-GBM disease were significantly higher than those in normal controls [114]. Although serum BAFF levels were not correlated with anti-GBM antibodies titers, those levels were associated with the percentage of glomeruli with crescents. Elevated serum BAFF levels were also demonstrated in patients with Graves' disease [115], autoimmune pancreatitis [116], myasthenia gravis [117], idiopathic thrombocytopenic purpura [118] and multiple sclerosis [119].

4. Anti-BAFF agents in autoimmune diseases

Several biologic drugs have recently been developed in an attempt to block the BAFF-BAFF receptors pathway: belimumab, atacicept, tabalumab and blisibimod. Belimumab is a human monoclonal antibody that antagonizes the effect of BAFF by binding to the free form of the cytokine [120]. Atacicept is a TACI-Fc fusion protein that binds to and blocks the receptor for both BAFF and APRIL [121]. It acts both in homotrimers and heterotrimers and results in diminished plasma cell survival and antibody production in mice and humans [121].

Tabalumab and blisibimod both block the two biologically active forms of BAFF; tabalumab is a human monoclonal antibody and blisibimod is a fusion polypeptide protein [122].

Animal models have shown that BAFF antagonists substantially delay the onset of disease in SLE-prone NZB/W mice [59, 123, 124] and prevent collagen-induced arthritis in DBA1 mice [125]. Clinical trials of anti-BAFF agents have also been performed as described below.

4.1. Belimumab

Belimumab was the first anti-BAFF drug to be evaluated in RA patients. In a phase II study, patients fulfilling the American College of Rheumatology (ACR) criteria for RA for equal to or greater than 1 year who had at least moderate disease activity while undergoing therapy with a stable disease-modifying antirheumatic drug (DMARD) and failed equal to or greater than 1 DMARD were randomly assigned to placebo or belimumab 1, 4, or 10 mg/kg treatment, administered intravenously (IV) on days 1, 14 and 28 and then every 4 weeks for 24 weeks ($n = 283$) [126]. The American College of Rheumatology 20% improvement criteria (ACR20) responder rates after 24 weeks of treatment with placebo and belimumab 1, 4 and 10 mg/kg, defined as the primary endpoint, were 15.9, 34.7, 25.4 and 28.2%, respectively, indicating relatively low efficacy of belimumab in this RA cohort [126]. This study was followed by an optional 24-week extension ($n = 237$) in which all patients received belimumab and patients received belimumab had an ACR20 response of 41% at 48 weeks [126].

Three major trials of belimumab in SLE have been reported. In a phase II study, patients with a SELENA-SLEDAI score equal to or greater than 4 ($n = 449$) were randomly assigned to belimumab (1, 4, or 10 mg/kg) or placebo in a 52-week trial [127]. There was no significant reduction in SELENA-SLEDAI scores from baseline; 19.5% in the combined belimumab group versus 17.2% in the placebo group. The median time to first SLE flare was 67 days in the combined belimumab group versus 83 days in the placebo group.

The BLISS-52 trial included 865 SLE patients with moderate-to-severe disease (SELENA-SLEDAI score equal to or greater than 6) and positive ANA and/or anti-dsDNA who were randomized to receive IV belimumab 1 mg/kg ($n = 289$) or 10 mg/kg ($n = 290$) or placebo ($n = 288$) [128]. Fifty-eight percent of the autoantibody-positive SLE patients in the 10 mg/kg belimumab group showed an improved systemic lupus erythematosus responder index (SRI) at week 52 versus 44% in the placebo group. In the patients treated with belimumab 1 mg/kg, 51% had an improved SRI value at week 52, which was also a significantly better response than placebo group. In addition, belimumab was shown to be well tolerated; it reduced disease activity and improved serologic activity, prevented flares and reduced corticosteroid use.

The BLISS-76 study was conducted in 819 patients who were randomized to receive IV belimumab 1 mg/kg ($n = 271$) or 10 mg/kg ($n = 273$) or placebo ($n = 275$) for 72 weeks [129]. The primary efficacy endpoint in this study was the same as the BLISS-52 trial and 43.2% of the SLE patients in the 10 mg/kg belimumab group were SRI responders versus 33.5% in the placebo group at 52 weeks, although at 76 weeks there was no significant difference in response rate among three treatment groups (response rates at week 76 were 32.4, 39.1 and 38.5% with placebo, 1 mg/kg belimumab and 10 mg/kg belimumab, respectively).

In a phase II open-label clinical trial of belimumab for SjS, a total of 30 SjS patients were treated with 10 mg/kg belimumab in weeks 0, 2 and 4 and every 4 weeks until week 24. The mean dryness, fatigue and pain visual analogue scale (VAS) values changed from 7.8 to 6.2 (p = 0.0021), 6.9 to 6.0 (p = 0.0606) and 4.6 to 4.7, respectively. However, there was no significant change in the salivary flow or the Schirmer's test score [130].

4.2. Atacicept

Similar to the outcome with belimumab, a Phase Ib study or 73 RA patients treated with six escalating doses of atacicept demonstrated good local and systemic tolerability to the drug. Patients received atacicept or placebo as single doses (70, 210, or 630 mg) or as repeated doses given at 2-week intervals (three doses of 70 mg, three doses of 210 mg, or seven doses of 420 mg), followed by 10 weeks of trial assessments, with a follow-up assessment at 3 months after the final dose [131]. Treatment-related decreases in immunoglobulin (particularly IgM) and RF levels were evident and a clear decrease in anticitrullinated protein antibodies was observed in the cohort that received seven doses of 420 mg [131]. However, further studies with atacicept did not demonstrate significant efficacy in RA patients with inadequate response to methotrexate (MTX) [132] or tumor necrosis factor antagonists [133].

In a 52-week Phase II/III study of atacicept in SLE, at screening (day 14), patients were started on a regimen of high-dose corticosteroid (the lesser of 0.8 mg/kg/day or 60 mg/day prednisone) and mycophenolate mofetil (MMF; 0.5 g twice daily, increased to a maximum of 1.5 g twice daily). From Day 1, atacicept (150 mg, subcutaneously, twice weekly for 4 weeks, then 150 mg weekly for a planned 48 weeks) was initiated with MMF along with a tapered dose of corticosteroid [134]. However, the trial was terminated after the enrollment of six patients, due to an unexpected decline in serum IgG and the occurrence of serious infections; three of four atacicept-treated patients developed serious infections in association with low IgG levels [134].

In another 52-week Phase II/III study, patients with moderate-to-severe SLE were randomized to atacicept 75 mg or atacicept 150 mg administered subcutaneously or placebo twice-weekly for 4 weeks, then weekly for 48 weeks [135]. Although there was no difference in flare rates or time to first flare between the atacicept 75 mg and placebo groups, flare rates in patients treated with atacicept 150 mg were decreased compared with placebo (flare rate 43 and 60%, respectively; odds ratio [OR]: 0.49) and atacicept 150 mg was associated with a significant delay in time to first flare (hazard ratio [HR]: 0.56) [135]. Both atacicept doses were associated with reductions in total immunoglobulin levels and anti-dsDNA antibodies and with increases in C3 and C4 levels [135]. However, enrollment in the atacicept 150 mg arm was discontinued prematurely due to two deaths.

4.3. Tabalumab

In a Phase II study of tabalumab in RA, patients who were naïve to biologic therapy received infusions of tabalumab (30, 60, or 160 mg) or placebo at weeks 0, 3 and 6 in combination with MTX and were evaluated for 24 weeks [136]. The percentages of patients achieving an ACR20 response at week 16 in the 30-mg, 60-mg and 160-mg groups were significantly greater than the percentage of patients achieving an ACR20 response in the placebo group (57.6, 67.6, 51.5 and 29.4%, respectively) [136]. In a Phase II dose-ranging study [137], RA patients on stable

MTX (*n* = 158) were randomized to receive 1, 3, 10, 30, 60, or 120 mg tabalumab or placebo subcutaneously every 4 weeks for 24 weeks. The observed ACR50 response rate was significantly higher with only the 120 mg dose versus placebo at week 12 (33.3 vs. 11.1%) and week 20 (33.3 vs. 8.3%), but not at week 24. The ACR20 response rate was significantly higher with 120 mg versus placebo at week 12 (66.7 vs. 33.3%) and week 24. No other dose was significantly different from placebo at any time point for ACR20, except 60 mg at week 4 (38.5 vs. 11.1%).

However, in a 52-week Phase III study that enrolled 1041 patients with moderate-to-severe RA despite ongoing MTX, the evaluation of subcutaneous tabalumab 120 mg every 4 weeks or 90 mg every 2 weeks versus placebo, there were no significant differences in ACR20 responses at week 24 among treatment groups [138]. Another Phase III trial (called the FLEX-O study) enrolled 1004 patients who received subcutaneous 120 mg tabalumab every 4 weeks, 90 mg tabalumab every 2 weeks, or placebo over 24 weeks with a loading dose double the planned dose (240 mg, 180 mg, or placebo) at baseline. No differences in the ACR20 response rates were observed at week 24 (34.4, 33.5 and 31.5%) or any other measures of efficacy across the treatment groups [139].

In another Phase III study, 456 patients with active RA were evaluated after 24-week treatment with subcutaneous tabalumab (120 mg every 4 weeks or 90 mg every 2 weeks) versus placebo, with loading doses (240 or 180 mg) at week 0. There was no significant difference in week 24 ACR20 responses among the three groups (17.6, 24.3 and 20.0%) per a nonresponder imputation analysis [140].

In a study of tabalumab in SLE, a total of 2288 SLE patients were randomized (*n* = 1164 in ILLUMINATE-1 and *n* = 1124 in ILLUMINATE-2) to receive tabalumab or placebo [141, 142]. In the ILLUMINATE-1 study, 1164 patients with moderate-to-severe SLE (SELENA-SLEDAI score equal to or greater than 6 at baseline) received subcutaneous injections of tabalumab or placebo, starting with a loading dose (240 mg) at week 0 and followed by 120 mg every 2 weeks (*n* = 387), 120 mg every 4 weeks (*n* = 389), or placebo (*n* = 388). Similar proportions of patients in each group achieved an SRI-5 response at week 52 (31.8, 35.2 and 29.3% placebo), but an SRI-5 response was achieved with 120 mg every 4 weeks (37.0 vs. 29.8% placebo), but not 120 mg every 2 weeks (34.1%) and significant reductions in anti-dsDNA antibodies, increases in C3 and C4 and reductions in total B cells and immunoglobulins were observed with tabalumab [141].

In the ILLUMINATE-2 study, 1124 patients with moderate-to-severe SLE (SELENA-SLEDAI score equal to or greater than 6 at baseline) received subcutaneous injections of tabalumab or placebo, starting with a loading dose (240 mg) at week 0 and followed by 120 mg every 2 weeks (*n* = 372), 120 mg every 4 weeks (*n* = 376), or placebo (*n* = 376). An SRI-5 response at week 52 was achieved in the 120-mg every 2 weeks regimen (38.4 vs. 27.7%, placebo), but not with the less-frequent 120 mg every 4 weeks regimen (34.8%) [142]. Anti-dsDNA levels decreased in both tabalumab groups as early as week 4 and continued to decrease, remaining well below baseline levels through week 52.

4.4. Blisibimod

In the phase Ia study of single-dose blisibimod, SLE patients with mild disease that was stable/inactive at baseline enrolled into one of seven dose cohorts: 0.1, 0.3, 1.0, or 3.0 mg/kg subcutaneous or 1.0, 3.0, or 6.0 mg/kg intravenous blisibimod and subjects were sequentially enrolled into one of four dose cohorts: 0.3, 1.0, or 3.0 mg/kg subcutaneous or 6.0 mg/kg intravenous in phase Ib study of multiple-dose blisibimod [143]. Blisibimod changed the constituency of the B-cell pool and single and multiple doses of blisibimod exhibited approximate dose-proportional pharmacokinetics across the dose range 1.0–6.0 mg/kg. The PEARL-SC study was a 24-week treatment, Phase IIb randomized trial of 547 SLE patients with moderate-to-severe disease (SELENA-SLEDAI) score equal to or greater than 6 at baseline) who received placebo or blisibimod at one of three dose levels in an evaluation of the efficacy and safety of blisibimod [144]. Although the SRI-5 response rates were not significantly improved in the pooled blisibimod groups compared with placebo, they were higher in the patients randomized to the highest dose of blisibimod (200 mg once-weekly) compared to the pooled placebo group at week 20. In the patients with protein:creatine ratios of 1–6 at baseline, significant reductions in proteinuria were observed with blisibimod. Significant changes in anti-dsDNA antibodies, complement C3 and C4 and reductions in B cells were observed with blisibimod treatment.

5. Conclusion

Based on the results of studies of autoimmune disorders in animal models of BAFF overexpression and the elevated levels of serum BAFF observed in patients with autoimmune diseases, it appears that BAFF may be associated with autoimmune processes and that BAFF may be a potential biomarker for disease activity in autoimmune diseases. BAFF may also be important as a therapeutic target in those diseases and several BAFF-neutralizing agents are currently undergoing clinical trials.

Acknowledgements

The authors declare no conflict of interest.

The authors thank Prof. M. Kobayashi (Dept. of Nephrology, Tokyo Medical University Ibaraki Medical Center, Ami, Japan), Prof. K. Yamagata (Dept. of Nephrology, University of Tsukuba, Tsukuba, Japan) and Prof. Y. Kanno (Dept. of Nephrology, Tokyo Medical University, Tokyo, Japan), for their helpful advice. We thank Dr. H. Maruyama, Dr. Y. Miyamoto, Dr. M. Takayasu and Dr. H. Shimohata (Dept. of Nephrology, Tokyo Medical University Ibaraki Medical Center, Ami, Japan) for their clinical assistance.

Author details

Kouichi Hirayama[1]* and Miho Nagai[2]

*Address all correspondence to: k-hira@tokyo-med.ac.jp

1 Department of Nephrology, Tokyo Medical University Ibaraki Medical Center, Japan

2 Department of Nephrology, Tokyo Medical University, Japan

References

[1] Mackay F, Schneider P, Rennert P, Browning J. BAFF AND APRIL: a tutorial on B cell survival. Annu Rev Immunol. 2003; 21: 231–64.

[2] Schneider P, MacKay F, Steiner V, Hofmann K, Bodmer JL, Holler N, Ambrose C, Lawton P, Bixler S, Acha-Orbea H, Valmori D, Romero P, Werner-Favre C, Zubler RH, Browning JL, Tschopp J. BAFF, a novel ligand of the tumor necrosis factor family, stimulates B cell growth. J Exp Med. 1999; 189(11): 1747–56.

[3] Jiang Y, Ohtsuji M, Abe M, Li N, Xiu Y, Wen S, Shirai T, Hirose S. Polymorphism and chromosomal mapping of the mouse gene for B-cell activating factor belonging to the tumor necrosis factor family (Baff) and association with the autoimmune phenotype. Immunogenetics. 2001; 53(9): 810–13.

[4] Abu-Rish EY, Amrani Y, Browning MJ. Toll-like receptor 9 activation induces expression of membrane-bound B-cell activating factor (BAFF) on human B cells and leads to increased proliferation in response to both soluble and membrane-bound BAFF. Rheumatology. 2013; 52(7): 1190–201.

[5] Liu Y, Xu L, Opalka N, Kappler J, Shu HB, Zhang G. Crystal structure of sTALL-1 reveals a virus-like assembly of TNF family ligands. Cell. 2002; 108(3): 383–94.

[6] Stohl W. Therapeutic targeting of the BAFF/APRIL axis in systemic lupus erythematosus. Expert Opin Ther Targets. 2014; 18(4): 473–89.

[7] Moore PA, Belvedere O, Orr A, Pieri K, LaFleur DW, Feng P, Soppet D, Charters M, Gentz R, Parmelee D, Li Y, Galperina O, Giri J, Roschke V, Nardelli B, Carrell J, Sosnovtseva S, Greenfield W, Ruben SM, Olsen HS, Fikes J, Hilbert DM. BLyS: member of the tumor necrosis factor family and B lymphocyte stimulator. Science. 1999; 285(5425): 260–3.

[8] Nardelli B, Belvedere O, Roschke V, Moore PA, Olsen HS, Migone TS, Sosnovtseva S, Carrell JA, Feng P, Giri JG, Hilbert DM. Synthesis and release of B-lymphocyte stimulator from myeloid cells. Blood. 2001; 97(1): 198–204.

[9] Scapini P, Nardelli B, Nadali G, Calzetti F, Pizzolo G, Montecucco C, Cassatella MA. G-CSF-stimulated neutrophils are a prominent source of functional BLyS. J Exp Med. 2003; 197(3): 297–302.

[10] Huard B, Arlettaz L, Ambrose C, Kindler V, Mauri D, Roosnek E, Tschopp J, Schneider P, French LE. BAFF production by antigen-presenting cells provides T cell co-stimulation. Int Immunol. 2004; 16(3): 467–75.

[11] Gorelik L, Gilbride K, Dobles M, Kalled SL, Zandman D, Scott ML. Normal B cell homeostasis requires B cell activation factor production by radiation-resistant cells. J Exp Med. 2003; 198(6): 937–45.

[12] Stadanlick JE, Cancro MP. BAFF and the plasticity of peripheral B cell tolerance. Curr Opin Immunol. 2008; 20(2): 158–61.

[13] O'Connor BP, Raman VS, Erickson LD, Cook WJ, Weaver LK, Ahonen C, Lin LL, Mantchev GT, Bram RJ, Noelle RJ. BCMA is essential for the survival of long-lived bone marrow plasma cells. J Exp Med. 2004; 199(1): 91–8.

[14] Novak AJ, Darce JR, Arendt BK, Harder B, Henderson K, Kindsvogel W, Gross JA, Greipp PR, Jelinek DF. Expression of BCMA, TACI and BAFF-R in multiple myeloma: a mechanism for growth and survival. Blood. 2004; 103(2): 689–94.

[15] Hahne M, Kataoka T, Schröter M, Hofmann K, Irmler M, Bodmer JL, Schneider P, Bornand T, Holler N, French LE, Sordat B, Rimoldi D, Tschopp J. APRIL, a new ligand of the tumor necrosis factor family, stimulates tumor cell growth. J Exp Med. 1998; 188(6): 1185–90.

[16] Kelly K, Manos E, Jensen G, Nadauld L, Jones DA. APRIL/TRDL-1, a tumor necrosis factor-like ligand, stimulates cell death. Cancer Res. 2000; 60(4): 1021–7.

[17] López-Fraga M, Fernández R, Albar JP, Hahne M. Biologically active APRIL is secreted following intracellular processing in the Golgi apparatus by furin convertase. EMBO Rep. 2001; 2(10): 945–51.

[18] Ingold K, Zumsteg A, Tardivel A, Huard B, Steiner QG, Cachero TG, Qiang F, Gorelik L, Kalled SL, Acha-Orbea H, Rennert PD, Tschopp J, Schneider P. Identification of proteoglycans as the APRIL-specific binding partners. J Exp Med. 2005; 201(9): 1375–83.

[19] Kimberley FC, van Bostelen L, Cameron K, Hardenberg G, Marquart JA, Hahne M, Medema JP. The proteoglycan (heparan sulfate proteoglycan) binding domain of APRIL serves as a platform for ligand multimerization and cross-linking. FASEB J. 2009; 23(5): 1584–95.

[20] Mackay F, Schneider P. TACI, an enigmatic BAFF/APRIL receptor, with new unappreciated biochemical and biological properties. Cytokine Growth Factor Rev. 2008; 19(3–4): 263–76.

[21] Bossen C, Cachero TG, Tardivel A, Ingold K, Willen L, Dobles M, Scott ML, Maquelin A, Belnoue E, Siegrist CA, Chevrier S, Acha-Orbea H, Leung H, Mackay F, Tschopp J, Schneider P. TACI, unlike BAFF-R, is solely activated by oligomeric BAFF and APRIL to support survival of activated B cells and plasmablasts. Blood. 2008; 111(3): 1004–12.

[22] Schiemann B, Gommerman JL, Vora K, Cachero TG, Shulga-Morskaya S, Dobles M, Frew E, Scott ML. An essential role for BAFF in the normal development of B cells through a BCMA-independent pathway. Science. 2001; 293(5537): 2111–4.

[23] Schneider P, Takatsuka H, Wilson A, Mackay F, Tardivel A, Lens S, Cachero TG, Finke D, Beermann F, Tschopp J. Maturation of marginal zone and follicular B cells requires B cell activating factor of the tumor necrosis factor family and is independent of B cell maturation antigen. J Exp Med. 2001; 194(11): 1691–7.

[24] Hildebrand JM, Luo Z, Manske MK, Price-Troska T, Ziesmer SC, Lin W, Hostager BS, Slager SL, Witzig TE, Ansell SM, Cerhan JR, Bishop GA, Novak AJ. A BAFF-R mutation associated with non-Hodgkin lymphoma alters TRAF recruitment and reveals new insights into BAFF-R signaling. J Exp Med. 2010; 207(12): 2569–79.

[25] Darce JR, Arendt BK, Wu X, Jelinek DF. Regulated expression of BAFF-binding receptors during human B cell differentiation. J Immunol. 2007; 179(11): 7276–86.

[26] Gras MP, Laâbi Y, Linares-Cruz G, Blondel MO, Rigaut JP, Brouet JC, Leca G, Haguenauer-Tsapis R, Tsapis A. BCMAp: an integral membrane protein in the Golgi apparatus of human mature B lymphocytes. Int Immunol. 1995; 7(7): 1093–106.

[27] Seshasayee D, Valdez P, Yan M, Dixit VM, Tumas D, Grewal IS. Loss of TACI causes fatal lymphoproliferation and autoimmunity, establishing TACI as an inhibitory BLyS receptor. Immunity. 2003; 18(2): 279–88.

[28] Avery DT, Kalled SL, Ellyard JI, Ambrose C, Bixler SA, Thien M, Brink R, Mackay F, Hodgkin PD, Tangye SG. BAFF selectively enhances the survival of plasmablasts generated from human memory B cells. J Clin Invest. 2003; 112(2): 286–97.

[29] Cancro MP. Peripheral B-cell maturation: the intersection of selection and homeostasis. Immunol Rev 2004; 197: 89–101.

[30] Varfolomeev E, Kischkel F, Martin F, Seshasayee D, Wang H, Lawrence D, Olsson C, Tom L, Erickson S, French D, Schow P, Grewal IS, Ashkenazi A. APRIL-deficient mice have normal immune system development. Mol Cell Biol. 2004; 24(3): 997–1006.

[31] Mohr E, Serre K, Manz RA, Cunningham AF, Khan M, Hardie DL, Bird R, MacLennan IC. Dendritic cells and monocyte/macrophages that create the IL-6/APRIL-rich lymph node microenvironments where plasmablasts mature. J Immunol. 2009; 182(4): 2113–23.

[32] Bossen C, Cachero TG, Tardivel A, Ingold K, Willen L, Dobles M, Scott ML, Maquelin A, Belnoue E, Siegrist CA, Chevrier S, Acha-Orbea H, Leung H, Mackay F, Tschopp J, Schneider P. TACI, unlike BAFF-R, is solely activated by oligomeric BAFF and APRIL to support survival of activated B cells and plasmablasts. Blood. 2008; 111(3): 1004–12.

[33] Shulga-Morskaya S, Dobles M, Walsh ME, Ng LG, MacKay F, Rao SP, Kalled SL, Scott ML. B cell-activating factor belonging to the TNF family acts through separate receptors to support B cell survival and T cell-independent antibody formation. J Immunol. 2004; 173(4): 2331–41.

[34] von Bülow GU, van Deursen JM, Bram RJ. Regulation of the T-independent humoral response by TACI. Immunity. 2001; 14(5): 573–82.

[35] Litinskiy MB, Nardelli B, Hilbert DM, He B, Schaffer A, Casali P, Cerutti A. DCs induce CD40-independent immunoglobulin class switching through BLyS and APRIL. Nat Immunol. 2002; 3(9): 822–9.

[36] Sakurai D, Hase H, Kanno Y, Kojima H, Okumura K, Kobata T. TACI regulates IgA production by APRIL in collaboration with HSPG. Blood. 2007; 109(7): 2961–7.

[37] Huard B, McKee T, Bosshard C, Durual S, Matthes T, Myit S, Donze O, Frossard C, Chizzolini C, Favre C, Zubler R, Guyot JP, Schneider P, Roosnek E. APRIL secreted by neutrophils binds to heparan sulfate proteoglycans to create plasma cell niches in human mucosa. J Clin Invest. 2008; 118(8): 2887–95.

[38] Boulé MW, Broughton C, Mackay F, Akira S, Marshak-Rothstein A, Rifkin IR. Toll-like receptor 9-dependent and -independent dendritic cell activation by chromatin-immunoglobulin G complexes. J Exp Med. 2004; 199(12): 1631–40.

[39] Treml LS, Carlesso G, Hoek KL, Stadanlick JE, Kambayashi T, Bram RJ, Cancro MP, Khan WN. TLR stimulation modifies BLyS receptor expression in follicular and marginal zone B cells. J Immunol. 2007; 178(12): 7531–9.

[40] Katsenelson N, Kanswal S, Puig M, Mostowski H, Verthelyi D, Akkoyunlu M. Synthetic CpG oligodeoxynucleotides augment BAFF- and APRIL-mediated immunoglobulin secretion. Eur J Immunol. 2007; 37(7): 1785–95.

[41] Groom JR, Fletcher CA, Walters SN, Grey ST, Watt SV, Sweet MJ, Smyth MJ, Mackay CR, Mackay F. BAFF and MyD88 signals promote a lupuslike disease independent of T cells. J Exp Med. 2007; 204(8): 1959–71.

[42] Acosta-Rodríguez EV, Craxton A, Hendricks DW, Merino MC, Montes CL, Clark EA, Gruppi A. BAFF and LPS cooperate to induce B cells to become susceptible to CD95/Fas-mediated cell death. Eur J Immunol. 2007; 37(4): 990–1000.

[43] Chan TD, Gardam S, Gatto D, Turner VM, Silke J, Brink R. In vivo control of B-cell survival and antigen-specific B-cell responses. Immunol Rev. 2010; 237(1): 90–103.

[44] Xie P, Kraus ZJ, Stunz LL, Bishop GA. Roles of TRAF molecules in B lymphocyte function. Cytokine Growth Factor Rev. 2008; 19(3–4): 199–207.

[45] Xu LG, Shu HB. TNFR-associated factor-3 is associated with BAFF-R and negatively regulates BAFF-R-mediated NF-kappa B activation and IL-10 production. J Immunol. 2002; 169(12): 6883–9.

[46] Ni CZ, Oganesyan G, Welsh K, Zhu X, Reed JC, Satterthwait AC, Cheng G, Ely KR. Key molecular contacts promote recognition of the BAFF receptor by TNF receptor-associated factor 3: implications for intracellular signaling regulation. J Immunol. 2004; 173(12): 7394–400.

[47] Mackay F, Woodcock SA, Lawton P, Ambrose C, Baetscher M, Schneider P, Tschopp J, Browning JL. Mice transgenic for BAFF develop lymphocytic disorders along with autoimmune manifestations. J Exp Med. 1999; 190(11): 1697–710.

[48] Grech AP, Amesbury M, Chan T, Gardam S, Basten A, Brink R. TRAF2 differentially regulates the canonical and noncanonical pathways of NF-kappaB activation in mature B cells. Immunity. 2004; 21(5): 629–42.

[49] Gardam S, Sierro F, Basten A, Mackay F, Brink R. TRAF2 and TRAF3 signal adapters act cooperatively to control the maturation and survival signals delivered to B cells by the BAFF receptor. Immunity. 2008; 28(3): 391–401.

[50] Xie P, Stunz LL, Larison KD, Yang B, Bishop GA. Tumor necrosis factor receptor-associated factor 3 is a critical regulator of B cell homeostasis in secondary lymphoid organs. Immunity. 2007; 27(2): 253–67.

[51] He B, Chadburn A, Jou E, Schattner EJ, Knowles DM, Cerutti A. Lymphoma B cells evade apoptosis through the TNF family members BAFF/BLyS and APRIL. J Immunol. 2004; 172(5): 3268–79.

[52] Xia XZ, Treanor J, Senaldi G, Khare SD, Boone T, Kelley M, Theill LE, Colombero A, Solovyev I, Lee F, McCabe S, Elliott R, Miner K, Hawkins N, Guo J, Stolina M, Yu G, Wang J, Delaney J, Meng SY, Boyle WJ, Hsu H. TACI is a TRAF-interacting receptor for TALL-1, a tumor necrosis factor family member involved in B cell regulation. J Exp Med. 2000; 192(1): 137–43.

[53] He B, Santamaria R, Xu W, Cols M, Chen K, Puga I, Shan M, Xiong H, Bussel JB, Chiu A, Puel A, Reichenbach J, Marodi L, Döffinger R, Vasconcelos J, Issekutz A, Krause J, Davies G, Li X, Grimbacher B, Plebani A, Meffre E, Picard C, Cunningham-Rundles C, Casanova JL, Cerutti A. The transmembrane activator TACI triggers immunoglobulin class switching by activating B cells through the adaptor MyD88. Nat Immunol. 2010; 11(9): 836–45.

[54] Xu S, Lam KP. B-cell maturation protein, which binds the tumor necrosis factor family members BAFF and APRIL, is dispensable for humoral immune responses. Mol Cell Biol. 2001; 21(12): 4067–74.

[55] Shu HB, Johnson H. B cell maturation protein is a receptor for the tumor necrosis factor family member TALL-1. Proc Natl Acad Sci USA. 2000; 97(16): 9156–61.

[56] Hatzoglou A, Roussel J, Bourgeade MF, Rogier E, Madry C, Inoue J, Devergne O, Tsapis A. TNF receptor family member BCMA (B cell maturation) associates with TNF receptor-associated factor (TRAF) 1, TRAF2 and TRAF3 and activates NF-kappa B, elk-1, c-Jun N-terminal kinase and p38 mitogen-activated protein kinase. J Immunol. 2000; 165(3): 1322–30.

[57] Belnoue E, Pihlgren M, McGaha TL, Tougne C, Rochat AF, Bossen C, Schneider P, Huard B, Lambert PH, Siegrist CA. APRIL is critical for plasmablast survival in the bone marrow and poorly expressed by early-life bone marrow stromal cells. Blood. 2008; 111(5): 2755–64.

[58] Gross JA, Dillon SR, Mudri S, Johnston J, Littau A, Roque R, Rixon M, Schou O, Foley KP, Haugen H, McMillen S, Waggie K, Schreckhise RW, Shoemaker K, Vu T, Moore M, Grossman A, Clegg CH. TACI-Ig neutralizes molecules critical for Bcell development and autoimmune disease. Impaired B cell maturation in mice lacking BLyS. Immunity. 2001; 15(2): 289–302.

[59] Thompson JS, Bixler SA, Qian F, Vora K, Scott ML, Cachero TG, Hession C, Schneider P, Sizing ID, Mullen C, Strauch K, Zafari M, Benjamin CD, Tschopp J, Browning JL, Ambrose C. BAFF-R, a newly identified TNF receptor that specifically interacts with BAFF. Science. 2001(5537); 293: 2108–11.

[60] Gross JA, Johnston J, Mudri S, Enselman R, Dillon SR, Madden K, Xu W, Parrish-Novak J, Foster D, Lofton-Day C, Moore M, Littau A, Grossman A, Haugen H, Foley K, Blumberg H, Harrison K, Kindsvogel W, Clegg CH. TACI and BCMA are receptors for a TNF homologue implicated in B-cell autoimmune disease. Nature. 2000; 404(6781): 995–99.

[61] Khare SD, Sarosi I, Xia XZ, McCabe S, Miner K, Solovyev I, Hawkins N, Kelley M, Chang D, Van G, Ross L, Delaney J, Wang L, Lacey D, Boyle WJ, Hsu H. Severe B cell hyperplasia and autoimmune disease in TALL-1 transgenic mice. Proc Natl Acad Sci USA. 2000; 97(7): 3370–5.

[62] Groom J, Kalled SL, Cutler AH, Olson C, Woodcock SA, Schneider P, Tschopp J, Cachero TG, Batten M, Wheway J, Mauri D, Cavill D, Gordon TP, Mackay CR, Mackay F. Association of BAFF/BLyS overexpression and altered B cell differentiation with Sjögren's syndrome. J Clin Invest. 2002; 109(1): 59–68.

[63] Batten M, Groom J, Cachero TG, Qian F, Schneider P, Tschopp J, Browning JL, Mackay F. BAFF mediates survival of peripheral immature B lymphocytes. J Exp Med. 2000; 192(10): 1453–66.

[64] Thien M, Phan TG, Gardam S, Amesbury M, Basten A, Mackay F, Brink R. Excess BAFF rescues self-reactive B cells from peripheral deletion and allows them to enter forbidden follicular and marginal zone niches. Immunity. 2004; 20(6): 785–98.

[65] Ding H, Wang L, Wu X, Yan J, He Y, Ni B, Gao W, Zhong X. Blockade of B-cell-activating factor suppresses lupus-like syndrome in autoimmune BXSB mice. J Cell Mol Med. 2010; 14(6B): 1717–25.

[66] Jacob CO, Pricop L, Putterman C, Koss MN, Liu Y, Kollaros M, Bixler SA, Ambrose CM, Scott ML, Stohl W. Paucity of clinical disease despite serological autoimmunity and kidney pathology in lupus-prone New Zealand mixed 2328 mice deficient in BAFF. J Immunol. 2006; 177(4): 2671–80.

[67] Jacob N, Guo S, Mathian A, Koss MN, Gindea S, Putterman C, Jacob CO, Stohl W. B Cell and BAFF dependence of IFN-α-exaggerated disease in systemic lupus erythematosus-prone NZM 2328 mice. J Immunol. 2011; 186(8): 4984–93.

[68] Warnatz K, Salzer U, Rizzi M, Fischer B, Gutenberger S, Böhm J, Kienzler AK, Pan-Hammarström Q, Hammarström L, Rakhmanov M, Schlesier M, Grimbacher B, Peter HH, Eibel H. B-cell activating factor receptor deficiency is associated with an adult-onset antibody deficiency syndrome in humans. Proc Natl Acad Sci U S A. 2009; 106(33): 13945–50.

[69] Zhang J, Roschke V, Baker KP, Wang Z, Alarcón GS, Fessler BJ, Bastian H, Kimberly RP, Zhou T. Cutting edge: a role for B lymphocyte stimulator in systemic lupus erythematosus. J Immunol. 2001; 166(1): 6–10.

[70] Cheema GS, Roschke V, Hilbert DM, Stohl W. Elevated serum B lymphocyte stimulator levels in patients with systemic immune-based rheumatic diseases. Arthritis Rheum. 2001; 44(6): 1313–9.

[71] Stohl W, Metyas S, Tan SM, Cheema GS, Oamar B, Xu D, Roschke V, Wu Y, Baker KP, Hilbert DM. B lymphocyte stimulator overexpression in patients with systemic lupus erythematosus: longitudinal observations. Arthritis Rheum. 2003; 48(12): 3475–86.

[72] Petri M, Stohl W, Chatham W, McCune WJ, Chevrier M, Ryel J, Recta V, Zhong J, Freimuth W. Association of plasma B lymphocyte stimulator levels and disease activity in systemic lupus erythematosus. Arthritis Rheum. 2008; 58(8): 2453–9.

[73] Collins CE, Gavin AL, Migone TS, Hilbert DM, Nemazee D, Stohl W. B lymphocyte stimulator (BLyS) isoforms in systemic lupus erythematosus: disease activity correlates better with blood leukocyte BLyS mRNA levels than with plasma BLyS protein levels. Arthritis Res Ther. 2006; 8(1):R6.

[74] Duan JH, Jiang Y, Mu H, Tang ZQ. Expression of BAFF and BR3 in patients with systemic lupus erythematosus. Braz J Med Biol Res. 2016; 49(3): e4853.

[75] Carter RH, Zhao H, Liu X, Pelletier M, Chatham W, Kimberly R, Zhou T. Expression and occupancy of BAFF-R on B cells in systemic lupus erythematosus. Arthritis Rheum. 2005; 52(12): 3943–54.

[76] Zhao LD, Li Y, Smith MF Jr, Wang JS, Zhang W, Tang FL, Tian XP, Wang HY, Zhang FC, Ba DN, He W, Zhang X. Expressions of BAFF/BAFF receptors and their correlation with disease activity in Chinese SLE patients. Lupus. 2010; 19(13): 1534–49.

[77] Cheng Y, Yan S, Zhao W, Huang Q, Lian L, Wei W. The effect of BLyS on the activity of peripheral B lymphocytes mediated by BLyS receptors in patients with systemic lupus erythematosus. Scand J Clin Lab Invest. 2013; 73(2): 141–7.

[78] Pers JO, Daridon C, Devauchelle V, Jousse S, Saraux A, Jamin C, Youinou P. BAFF overexpression is associated with autoantibody production in autoimmune diseases. Ann N Y Acad Sci. 2005; 1050: 34–9.

[79] Bosello S, Youinou P, Daridon C, Tolusso B, Bendaoud B, Pietrapertosa D, Morelli A, Ferraccioli G. Concentrations of BAFF correlate with autoantibody levels, clinical disease activity and response to treatment in early rheumatoid arthritis. J Rheumatol. 2008; 35(7): 1256–64.

[80] Tan SM, Xu D, Roschke V, Perry JW, Arkfeld DG, Ehresmann GR, Migone TS, Hilbert DM, Stohl W. Local production of B lymphocyte stimulator protein and APRIL in arthritic joints of patients with inflammatory arthritis. Arthritis Rheum. 2003; 48(4): 982–92.

[81] Nakajima K, Itoh K, Nagatani K, Okawa-Takatsuji M, Fujii T, Kuroki H, Katsuragawa Y, Aotsuka S, Mimori A. Expression of BAFF and BAFF-R in the synovial tissue of patients with rheumatoid arthritis. Scand J Rheumatol. 2007; 36(5): 365–72.

[82] Ohata J, Zvaifler NJ, Nishio M, Boyle DL, Kalled SL, Carson DA, Kipps TJ. Fibroblast-like synoviocytes of mesenchymal origin express functional B cell-activating factor of the TNF family in response to proinflammatory cytokines. J Immunol. 2005; 174(2): 864–70.

[83] Rochas C, Hillion S, Saraux A, Mageed RA, Youinou P, Jamin C, Devauchelle V. Transmembrane BAFF from rheumatoid synoviocytes requires interleukin-6 to induce the expression of recombination-activating gene in B lymphocytes. Arthritis Rheum. 2009; 60(5): 1261–71.

[84] Alsaleh G, François A, Knapp AM, Schickel JN, Sibilia J, Pasquali JL, Gottenberg JE, Wachsmann D, Soulas-Sprauel P. Synovial fibroblasts promote immunoglobulin class switching by a mechanism involving BAFF. Eur J Immunol. 2011; 41(7): 2113–22.

[85] de la Torre I, Moura RA, Leandro MJ, Edwards J, Cambridge G. B-cell-activating factor receptor expression on naïve and memory B cells: relationship with relapse in patients with rheumatoid arthritis following B-cell depletion therapy. Ann Rheum Dis. 2010; 69(12): 2181–8.

[86] Woo YJ, Yoon BY, Jhun JY, Oh HJ, Min SW, Cho ML, Park SH, Kim HY, Min JK. Regulation of B cell activating factor (BAFF) receptor expression by NF-KB signaling in rheumatoid arthritis B cells. Exp Mol Med. 2011 30; 43(6): 350–7.

[87] Moura RA, Canhão H, Polido-Pereira J, Rodrigues AM, Navalho M, Mourão AF, Resende C, Campanilho-Marques R, Madruga Dias J, da Silva JA, Graca L, Fonseca JE. BAFF and TACI gene expression are increased in patients with untreated very early rheumatoid arthritis. J Rheumatol. 2013; 40(8): 1293–302.

[88] Jonsson MV, Szodoray P, Jellestad S, Jonsson R, Skarstein K. Association between circulating levels of the novel TNF family members APRIL and BAFF and lymphoid organization in primary Sjögren's syndrome. J Clin Immunol. 2005; 25(3): 189–201.

[89] Mariette X, Roux S, Zhang J, Bengoufa D, Lavie F, Zhou T, Kimberly R. The level of BLyS (BAFF) correlates with the titre of autoantibodies in human Sjögren's syndrome. Ann Rheum Dis. 2003; 62(2): 168–71.

[90] Candon S, Gottenberg JE, Bengoufa D, Chatenoud L, Mariette X. Quantitative assessment of antibodies to ribonucleoproteins in primary Sjögren syndrome: correlation with B-cell biomarkers and disease activity. Ann Rheum Dis. 2009; 68(7): 1208–12.

[91] Szodoray P, Jellestad S, Alex P, Zhou T, Wilson PC, Centola M, Brun JG, Jonsson R. Programmed cell death of peripheral blood B cells determined by laser scanning cytometry in Sjögren's syndrome with a special emphasis on BAFF. J Clin Immunol. 2004; 24(6): 600–11.

[92] Szodoray P, Alex P, Jonsson MV, Knowlton N, Dozmorov I, Nakken B, Delaleu N, Jonsson R, Centola M. Distinct profiles of Sjögren's syndrome patients with ectopic salivary gland germinal centers revealed by serum cytokines and BAFF. Clin Immunol. 2005; 117(2): 168–76.

[93] Lavie F, Miceli-Richard C, Ittah M, Sellam J, Gottenberg JE, Mariette X. B-cell activating factor of the tumor necrosis factor family expression in blood monocytes and T cells from patients with primary Sjögren's syndrome. Scand J Immunol. 2008; 67(2): 185–92.

[94] Lavie F, Miceli-Richard C, Quillard J, Roux S, Leclerc P, Mariette X. Expression of BAFF (BLyS) in T cells infiltrating labial salivary glands from patients with Sjögren's syndrome. J Pathol. 2004; 202(4): 496–502.

[95] Ittah M, Miceli-Richard C, Eric Gottenberg J, Lavie F, Lazure T, Ba N, Sellam J, Lepajolec C, Mariette X. B cell-activating factor of the tumor necrosis factor family (BAFF) is expressed under stimulation by interferon in salivary gland epithelial cells in primary Sjögren's syndrome. Arthritis Res Ther. 2006; 8(2): R51.

[96] Daridon C, Devauchelle V, Hutin P, Le Berre R, Martins-Carvalho C, Bendaoud B, Dueymes M, Saraux A, Youinou P, Pers JO. Aberrant expression of BAFF by B lymphocytes infiltrating the salivary glands of patients with primary Sjögren's syndrome. Arthritis Rheum. 2007; 56(4): 1134–44.

[97] Yoshimoto K, Tanaka M, Kojima M, Setoyama Y, Kameda H, Suzuki K, Tsuzaka K, Ogawa Y, Tsubota K, Abe T, Takeuchi T. Regulatory mechanisms for the production of BAFF and IL-6 are impaired in monocytes of patients of primary Sjögren's syndrome. Arthritis Res Ther. 2011; 13(5): R170.

[98] Sellam J, Miceli-Richard C, Gottenberg JE, Ittah M, Lavie F, Lacabaratz C, Gestermann N, Proust A, Lambotte O, Mariette X. Decreased B cell activating factor receptor expression on peripheral lymphocytes associated with increased disease activity in primary Sjögren's syndrome and systemic lupus erythematosus. Ann Rheum Dis. 2007; 66(6): 790–7.

[99] Quartuccio L, Fabris M, Moretti M, Barone F, Bombardieri M, Rupolo M, Lombardi S, Pitzalis C, Beltrami CA, Curcio F, De Vita S. Resistance to rituximab therapy and local BAFF overexpression in Sjögren's syndrome-related myoepithelial sialadenitis and low-grade parotid B-cell lymphoma. Open Rheumatol J. 2008; 2: 38–43.

[100] Nezos A, Papageorgiou A, Fragoulis G, Ioakeimidis D, Koutsilieris M, Tzioufas AG, Moutsopoulos HM, Voulgarelis M, Mavragani CP. B-cell activating factor genetic variants in lymphomagenesis associated with primary Sjogren's syndrome. J Autoimmun. 2014; 51: 89–98.

[101] Papageorgiou A, Mavragani CP, Nezos A, Zintzaras E, Quartuccio L, De Vita S, Koutsilieris M, Tzioufas AG, Moutsopoulos HM, Voulgarelis M. A BAFF receptor His159Tyr mutation in Sjögren's syndrome-related lymphoproliferation. Arthritis Rheumatol. 2015; 67(10): 2732–41.

[102] Krumbholz M, Specks U, Wick M, Kalled SL, Jenne D, Meinl E. BAFF is elevated in serum of patients with Wegener's granulomatosis. J Autoimmun. 2005; 25(4): 298–302.

[103] Sanders JS, Huitma MG, Kallenberg CG, Stegeman CA. Plasma levels of soluble interleukin 2 receptor, soluble CD30, interleukin 10 and B cell activator of the tumour necrosis factor family during follow-up in vasculitis associated with proteinase 3-antineutrophil cytoplasmic antibodies: associations with disease activity and relapse. Ann Rheum Dis. 2006; 65(11): 1484–9.

[104] Bader L, Koldingsnes W, Nossent J. B-lymphocyte activating factor levels are increased in patients with Wegener's granulomatosis and inversely correlated with ANCA titer. Clin Rheumatol. 2010; 29(9): 1031–5.

[105] Schneeweis C, Rafalowicz M, Feist E, Buttgereit F, Rudolph PE, Burmester GR, Egerer K. Increased levels of BLyS and sVCAM-1 in anti-neutrophil cytoplasmatic antibody (ANCA)-associated vasculitides (AAV). Clin Exp Rheumatol. 2010; 28(1 Suppl 57): 62–6.

[106] Nagai M, Hirayama K, Ebihara I, Shimohata H, Kobayashi M, Koyama A. Serum levels of BAFF and APRIL in myeloperoxidase anti-neutrophil cytoplasmic autoantibody-associated renal vasculitis: association with disease activity. Nephron Clin Pract. 2011; 118(4): c339–45.

[107] Xin G, Chen M, Su Y, Xu LX, Zhao MH, Li KS. Serum B-cell activating factor in myeloperoxiase-antineutrophil cytoplasmic antibodies-associated vasculitis. Am J Med Sci. 2014; 348(1): 25–9.

[108] Holden NJ, Williams JM, Morgan MD, Challa A, Gordon J, Pepper RJ, Salama AD, Harper L, Savage CO. ANCA-stimulated neutrophils release BLyS and promote B cell survival: a clinically relevant cellular process. Ann Rheum Dis. 2011; 70(12): 2229–33.

[109] Abdulahad WH, Lepse N, Stegeman CA, Huitema MG, Doornbos-van der Meer B, Tadema H, Rutgers A, Limburg PC, Kallenberg CG, Heeringa P. Increased frequency of circulating IL-21 producing Th-cells in patients with granulomatosis with polyangiitis (GPA). Arthritis Res Ther. 2013; 15(3): R70.

[110] Lepse N, Land J, Rutgers A, Kallenberg CG, Stegeman CA, Abdulahad WH, Heeringa P. Toll-like receptor 9 activation enhances B cell activating factor and interleukin-21 induced anti-proteinase 3 autoantibody production in vitro. Rheumatology (Oxford). 2016; 55(1): 162–72.

[111] Nagai M, Hirayama K, Ebihara I, Kobayashi M. Serum soluble levels of the transmembrane activator and calcium-modulator and cyclophilin-ligand interactor in MPO-ANCA-associated renal vasculitis. Clin Exp Nephrol. 2015; 19(4): 759–60.

[112] Zhao Y, Odell E, Choong LM, Barone F, Fields P, Wilkins B, Tungekar FM, Patel P, Sanderson JD, Sangle S, D'Cruz D, Spencer J. Granulomatosis with polyangiitis involves sustained mucosal inflammation that is rich in B-cell survival factors and autoantigen. Rheumatology. 2012; 51(9): 1580–6.

[113] Mueller A, Brieske C, Schinke S, Csernok E, Gross WL, Hasselbacher K, Voswinkel J, Holl-Ulrich K. Plasma cells within granulomatous inflammation display signs pointing to autoreactivity and destruction in granulomatosis with polyangiitis. Arthritis Res Ther. 2014; 6(1): R55.

[114] Xin G, Cui Z, Su Y, Xu LX, Zhao MH, Li KS. Serum BAFF and APRIL might be associated with disease activity and kidney damage in patients with anti-glomerular basement membrane disease. Nephrology. 2013; 18(3): 209–14.

[115] Vannucchi G, Covelli D, Currò N, Dazzi D, Maffini A, Campi I, Bonara P, Guastella C, Pignataro L, Ratiglia R, Beck-Peccoz P, Salvi M. Serum BAFF concentrations in patients with Graves' disease and orbitopathy before and after immunosuppressive therapy. J Clin Endocrinol Metab. 2012; 97(5): E755–9.

[116] Yamanishi H, Kumagi T, Yokota T, Azemoto N, Koizumi M, Kobayashi Y, Abe M, Murakami H, Hiasa Y, Matsuura B, Kawamoto H, Yamamoto K, Onji M. Clinical significance of B cell-activating factor in autoimmune pancreatitis. Pancreas. 2011; 40(6): 840–5.

[117] Kim JY, Yang Y, Moon JS, Lee EY, So SH, Lee HS, Park KD, Choi YC. Serum BAFF expression in patients with myasthenia gravis. J Neuroimmunol. 2008; 199(1–2): 151–4.

[118] Zhou Z, Chen Z, Li H, Chen X, Xu J, Gu D, Du W, Zheng C, Zhang L, Huang Y, Ren Q, Yang R. BAFF and BAFF-R of peripheral blood and spleen mononuclear cells in idiopathic thrombocytopenic purpura. Autoimmunity. 2009; 42(2): 112–9.

[119] Thangarajh M, Gomes A, Masterman T, Hillert J, Hjelmström P. Expression of B-cell-activating factor of the TNF family (BAFF) and its receptors in multiple sclerosis. J Neuroimmunol. 2004; 152(1–2): 183–90.

[120] Halpern WG, Lappin P, Zanardi T, Cai W, Corcoran M, Zhong J, Baker KP. Chronic administration of belimumab, a BLyS antagonist, decreases tissue and peripheral blood B-lymphocyte populations in cynomolgus monkeys: pharmacokinetic, pharmacodynamic and toxicologic effects. Toxicol Sci. 2006; 91(2): 586–99.

[121] Munafo A, Priestley A, Nestorov I, Visich J, Rogge M. Safety, pharmacokinetics and pharmacodynamics of atacicept in healthy volunteers. Eur J Clin Pharmacol. 2007; 63(7): 647–56.

[122] Stohl W. Biologic differences between various inhibitors of the BLyS/BAFF pathway: should we expect differences between belimumab and other inhibitors in development? Curr Rheumatol Rep. 2012; 14(4): 303–9.

[123] Ramanujam M, Wang X, Huang W, Schiffer L, Grimaldi C, Akkerman A, Diamond B, Madaio MP, Davidson A. Mechanism of action of transmembrane activator and calcium modulator ligand interactor-Ig in murine systemic lupus erythematosus. J Immunol. 2004; 173(5): 3524–34.

[124] Kayagaki N, Yan M, Seshasayee D, Wang H, Lee W, French DM, Grewal IS, Cochran AG, Gordon NC, Yin J, Starovasnik MA, Dixit VM. BAFF/BLyS receptor 3 binds the B cell survival factor BAFF ligand through a discrete surface loop and promotes processing of NF-kappaB2. Immunity. 2002; 17(4): 515–24.

[125] Wang H, Marsters SA, Baker T, Chan B, Lee WP, Fu L, Tumas D, Yan M, Dixit VM, Ashkenazi A, Grewal IS. TACI-ligand interactions are required for T cell activation and collagen-induced arthritis in mice. Nat Immunol. 2001; 2(7): 632–7.

[126] Stohl W, Merrill JT, McKay JD, Lisse JR, Zhong ZJ, Freimuth WW, Genovese MC. Efficacy and safety of belimumab in patients with rheumatoid arthritis: a phase II, randomized, double-blind, placebo-controlled, dose-ranging Study. J Rheumatol. 2013; 40(5): 579–89.

[127] Wallace DJ, Stohl W, Furie RA, Lisse JR, McKay JD, Merrill JT, Petri MA, Ginzler EM, Chatham WW, McCune WJ, Fernandez V, Chevrier MR, Zhong ZJ, Freimuth WW. A phase II, randomized, double-blind, placebo-controlled, dose-ranging study of belimumab in patients with active systemic lupus erythematosus. Arthritis Rheum. 2009; 61(9): 1168–78.

[128] Navarra SV, Guzmán RM, Gallacher AE, Hall S, Levy RA, Jimenez RE, Li EK, Thomas M, Kim HY, León MG, Tanasescu C, Nasonov E, Lan JL, Pineda L, Zhong ZJ, Freimuth W, Petri MA. BLISS-52 Study Group. Efficacy and safety of belimumab in patients with active systemic lupus erythematosus: a randomised, placebo-controlled, phase 3 trial. Lancet. 2011; 377(9767): 721–31.

[129] Furie R, Petri M, Zamani O, Cervera R, Wallace DJ, Tegzová D, Sanchez-Guerrero J, Schwarting A, Merrill JT, Chatham WW, Stohl W, Ginzler EM, Hough DR, Zhong ZJ, Freimuth W, van Vollenhoven RF. BLISS-76 Study Group. A phase III, randomized, placebo-controlled study of belimumab, a monoclonal antibody that inhibits B lymphocyte stimulator, in patients with systemic lupus erythematosus. Arthritis Rheum. 2011; 63(12): 3918–30.

[130] Mariette X, Seror R, Quartuccio L, Baron G, Salvin S, Fabris M, Desmoulins F, Nocturne G, Ravaud P, De Vita S. Efficacy and safety of belimumab in primary Sjögren's syndrome: results of the BELISS open-label phase II study. Ann Rheum Dis. 2015; 74(3): 526–31.

[131] Tak PP, Thurlings RM, Rossier C, Nestorov I, Dimic A, Mircetic V, Rischmueller M, Nasonov E, Shmidt E, Emery P, Munafo A. Atacicept in patients with rheumatoid arthritis: results of a multicenter, phase Ib, double-blind, placebo-controlled, dose-escalating, single- and repeated-dose study. Arthritis Rheum. 2008; 58(1): 61–72.

[132] van Vollenhoven RF, Kinnman N, Vincent E, Wax S, Bathon J. Atacicept in patients with rheumatoid arthritis and an inadequate response to methotrexate: results of a phase II, randomized, placebo-controlled trial. Arthritis Rheum. 2011; 63(7): 1782–92.

[133] Genovese MC, Kinnman N, de La Bourdonnaye G, Pena Rossi C, Tak PP. Atacicept in patients with rheumatoid arthritis and an inadequate response to tumor necrosis factor antagonist therapy: results of a phase II, randomized, placebo-controlled, dose-finding trial. Arthritis Rheum. 2011; 63(7): 1793–803.

[134] Ginzler EM, Wax S, Rajeswaran A, Copt S, Hillson J, Ramos E, Singer NG. Atacicept in combination with MMF and corticosteroids in lupus nephritis: results of a prematurely terminated trial. Arthritis Res Ther. 2012 7; 14(1): R33.

[135] Isenberg D, Gordon C, Licu D, Copt S, Rossi CP, Wofsy D. Efficacy and safety of atacicept for prevention of flares in patients with moderate-to-severe systemic lupus erythematosus (SLE): 52-week data (APRIL-SLE randomised trial). Ann Rheum Dis. 2015; 74(11): 2006–15.

[136] Genovese MC, Bojin S, Biagini IM, Mociran E, Cristei D, Mirea G, Georgescu L, Sloan-Lancaster J. Tabalumab in rheumatoid arthritis patients with an inadequate response to methotrexate and naïve to biologic therapy: a phase II, randomized, placebo-controlled trial. Arthritis Rheum. 2013; 65(4): 880–9.

[137] Genovese MC, Lee E, Satterwhite J, Veenhuizen M, Disch D, Berclaz PY, Myers S, Sides G, Benichou O. A phase 2 dose-ranging study of subcutaneous tabalumab for the treatment of patients with active rheumatoid arthritis and an inadequate response to methotrexate. Ann Rheum Dis. 2013; 72(9): 1453–60.

[138] Smolen JS, Weinblatt ME, van der Heijde D, Rigby WF, van Vollenhoven R, Bingham CO 3rd, Veenhuizen M, Gill A, Zhao F, Komocsar WJ, Berclaz PY, Ortmann R, Lee C. Efficacy and safety of tabalumab, an anti-B-cell-activating factor monoclonal antibody, in patients with rheumatoid arthritis who had an inadequate response to methotrexate therapy: results from a phase III multicentre, randomised, double-blind study. Ann Rheum Dis. 2015; 74(8): 1567–70.

[139] Genovese MC, Silverman GJ, Emery P, Gupta RC, Gill A, Veenhuizen M, Xie L, Komocsar WJ, Berclaz PY, Lee C. Efficacy and safety of tabalumab, an anti-B-cell-activating factor monoclonal antibody, in a heterogeneous rheumatoid arthritis population: results from a randomized, placebo-controlled, phase 3 trial (FLEX-O). J Clin Rheumatol. 2015; 21(5): 231–8.

[140] Schiff M, Combe B, Dörner T, Kremer JM, Huizinga TW, Veenhuizen M, Gill A, Komocsar W, Berclaz PY, Ortmann R, Lee C. Efficacy and safety of tabalumab, an anti-BAFF monoclonal antibody, in patients with moderate-to-severe rheumatoid arthritis and inadequate response to TNF inhibitors: results of a randomised, double-blind, placebo-controlled, phase 3 study. RMD Open. 2015; 1(1): e000037.

[141] Isenberg DA, Petri M, Kalunian K, Tanaka Y, Urowitz MB, Hoffman RW, Morgan-Cox M, Iikuni N, Silk M, Wallace DJ. Efficacy and safety of subcutaneous tabalumab in patients with systemic lupus erythematosus: results from ILLUMINATE-1, a 52-week, phase III, multicentre, randomised, double-blind, placebo-controlled study. Ann Rheum Dis. 2016; 75(2): 323–31.

[142] Merrill JT, van Vollenhoven RF, Buyon JP, Furie RA, Stohl W, Morgan-Cox M, Dickson C anderson PW, Lee C, Berclaz PY, Dörner T. Efficacy and safety of subcutaneous tabalumab, a monoclonal antibody to B-cell activating factor, in patients with systemic lupus erythematosus: results from ILLUMINATE-2, a 52-week, phase III, multicentre, randomised, double-blind, placebo-controlled study. Ann Rheum Dis. 2016; 75(2): 332–40.

[143] Stohl W, Merrill JT, Looney RJ, Buyon J, Wallace DJ, Weisman MH, Ginzler EM, Cooke B, Holloway D, Kaliyaperumal A, Kuchimanchi KR, Cheah TC, Rasmussen E, Ferbas J, Belouski SS, Tsuji W, Zack DJ. Treatment of systemic lupus erythematosus patients with the BAFF antagonist "peptibody" blisibimod (AMG 623/A-623): results from randomized, double-blind phase 1a and phase 1b trials. Arthritis Res Ther. 2015 20; 17: 215.

[144] Furie RA, Leon G, Thomas M, Petri MA, Chu AD, Hislop C, Martin RS, Scheinberg MA; PEARL-SC Study. A phase 2, randomised, placebo-controlled clinical trial of blisibimod, an inhibitor of B cell activating factor, in patients with moderate-to-severe systemic lupus erythematosus, the PEARL-SC study. Ann Rheum Dis. 2015; 74(9): 1667–75.